The Volumetrics
Weight-Control Plan

The Volumetrics Weight-Control Plan

Feel Full on Fewer Calories

Barbara Rolls, Ph.D., and Robert A. Barnett

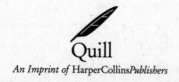

Quill

An Imprint of HarperCollinsPublishers

A hardcover edition of this book was published in 2000 by HarperCollins Publishers.

THE VOLUMETRICS WEIGHT-CONTROL PLAN. Copyright © 2000 by Barbara Rolls and Robert A. Barnett. All rights reserved. Printed in the United States of America. No part of this book may be used or reproduced in any manner whatsoever without written permission except in the case of brief quotations embodied in critical articles and reviews. For information address HarperCollins Publishers Inc., 10 East 53rd Street, New York, NY 10022.

HarperCollins books may be purchased for educational, business, or sales promotional use. For information please write: Special Markets Department, HarperCollins Publishers Inc., 10 East 53rd Street, New York, NY 10022.

First Quill edition published 2000.

Designed by Joel Avirom & Jason Snyder
Illustrations by Laura Hartman Maestro

Library of Congress Cataloging-in-Publication Data is available.

ISBN 0-06-093272-4

01 02 03 04 ❖/RRD 10 9 8 7 6 5 4 3 2

*To the staff and students in the Eating Lab
and to the many participants in our studies
who have helped us to understand why people eat*

Contents

Acknowledgments

MUCH IN THIS BOOK DEPENDS on the thoughtful comments and extensive analyses of foods and recipes by Elizabeth (Liz) Bell, a Ph.D. student in the Eating Lab at Penn State. She has also been involved in the critical studies of energy density that form the scientific basis of this book. Harry Rice, another Ph.D. student in nutrition at Penn State, has been by her side calculating whatever needs to be calculated.

We are indebted to Debby Maugans Nakos of Southern Food Consultants in Birmingham, Alabama, for making our ideas delicious with her stylish, practical recipes, and her help with the menu plans. For the illustrations, we were very lucky to have found Laura H. Maestro in New York City, whose drawings are both accurate and lovely.

For her appreciation of the potential of this new approach to weight management, and her sharp editing skills that kept us on message, we thank our editor, Susan Friedland. We are indebted to our agent, Alice Martell, of The Martell Group in New York City, for her early enthusiasm for this project, and her trustworthy counsel through all phases of the project.

We thank Joan Conway, Maureen Mackey, Christine Pelkman, Liane Roe, Madeleine Sigman-Grant, Marion Nestle, and Larry Lindner for their suggestions on ways to improve the messages and the nutritional information in the book.

Barbara Rolls thanks the National Institutes of Health, Institute of Diabetes and Digestive and Kidney Diseases for funding the research that led to this book. She is grateful to Penn State for providing such an excellent and congenial environment for conducting research. She thanks family, friends, and colleagues for being supportive while the book was being written. Finally, she thanks Charlie Brueggebors for keeping her going on delicious *Volumetric* meals.

Robert A. Barnett thanks his wife, Chris, for her love and support that has yet again kept him safe and sound through an unruly book project, and for taking caring of Emily on those late nights. I owe you a cottage.

Both authors thank the following colleagues who generously offered their time to discuss their professional insights with us:

David J. Baer, Ph.D., Research Physiologist, U.S. Department of Agriculture, Human Nutrition Research Center, Beltsville, Maryland; Leann L. Birch, Professor and Department Head, Human Development and Family Studies, Penn State University, University Park; Steven Blair, PED, Director of Research, Cooper Institute, Dallas, Texas; Terry Brownlee, M.Ph., R.D., Nutrition Director at the Duke University Diet & Fitness Center, Durham, North Carolina; Tim Byers, M.D., M.Ph., Professor of Preventive Medicine, University of Colorado School of Medicine, Denver, Colorado; Adam Drewnowski, Ph.D., Director of Nutritional Sciences, University of Washington, Seattle; Miles Faith, Ph.D., Research Scientist, Obesity Research Center, St. Lukes Roosevelt Hospital, New York, New York; Richard W. Foltin, Ph.D., Associate Professor of Behavioral Biology, College of Physicians and Surgeons, Columbia University, New York, New York; John Foreyt, Ph.D., Director of the Nutrition Research Clinic, Baylor University, Houston, Texas; James O. Hill, Ph.D., Professor of Pediatrics and Medicine, University of Colorado Health Sciences Center, Denver; Marsha Hudnall, M.S., R.D., Director of Nutrition, Green Mountain at Fox Run, Ludlow, Vermont; David Jenkins, M.D., Professor of Nutrition, University of Toronto, Canada; Jeanne Jones, *Cook It Light* columnist; Mary Abbot Hess, L.H.D., R.D., of Hess & Hunt in Chicago, Illinois; Barbara Kafka, author of *Soup: A Way of Life*; Georgia Kostas, Ph.D., Director of Nutrition, Cooper Clinic, Dallas, Texas; Nancy Keim, Ph.D., R.D., Research Nutrition Scientist, U.S. Department of Agriculture, Human Nutrition Research Center, Davis, California; Susan M. Kleiner, Ph.D., R.D., Assistant Professor in Nutritional Sciences, University of Washington, Seattle; Mary Lou Klem, Ph.D., Senior Research Fellow, University of Pittsburgh School of Medicine, Pittsburgh, Pennsylvania; Kenneth Koch, M.D., Professor of Medicine, Department of Gastroenterology, Penn State University College of Medicine, Hershey; Penny Kris-Etherton, Ph.D., Distinguished Professor of Nutrition, Penn State University, University Park; Alan Kristal, Ph.D., Member, the Cancer Prevention Research Program, Fred Hutchinson Cancer Research Center, Seattle, Washington; Larry Lindner, Editor of the *Tufts Health & Nutrition Letter* in Boston, Massachusetts; Judith Marlett, Ph.D., R.D., Professor of Nutritional Sciences, University of

Wisconsin-Madison; Megan McCrory, Ph.D., Post-Doctoral Research Associate, U.S. Department of Agriculture, Research Center on Aging, Tufts University, Boston, Massachusetts; Karen Miller-Kovachs, M.S., R.D., lead scientist at Weight Watchers International; Kathleen J. Motil, M.D., Ph.D., Assistant Professor of Pediatrics, Baylor College of Medicine, Houston, Texas; Linda Nebling, Ph.D., M.Ph., R.D., Nutritionist, National Cancer Institute, Washington, D.C.; Marion Nestle, Ph.D., M.Ph., Chair, Department of Nutrition and Food Studies, New York University, New York; Elizabeth Pivonka, Ph.D., R.D., President, Produce for Better Health Foundation, Wilmington, Delaware; Janet Polivy, Ph.D., Professor of Psychology, University of Toronto, Mississauga, Ontario, Canada; Barry Popkin, Ph.D., Professor of Nutrition, University of North Carolina, Chapel Hill; Gerald Reaven, M.D., Professor of Medicine, Stanford University School of Medicine, Palo Alto, California; Peter Reeds, Ph.D., Professor of Pediatrics, Baylor College of Medicine, Houston, Texas; Eric Rimm, Ph.D., Associate Professor of Epidemiology and Nutrition, Harvard School of Public Health, Boston, Massachusetts; Susan B. Roberts, Ph.D., Director, Energy Metabolism Laboratory, U.S. Department of Agriculture, Research Center on Aging, Tufts University, Boston, Massachusetts; Paul Rozin, Ph.D., Professor of Psychology, University of Pennsylvania, Philadelphia; Barbara Schneeman, Ph.D., Professor of Nutrition, University of California, Davis; Judith Stern, Ph.D., Professor of Nutrition, University of California, Davis; Angelo Tremblay, Ph.D., Professor of Nutrition and Physiology, Laval University, Ste-Foy, Quebec, Canada; Brian Wansink, Ph.D., Professor of Marketing and Consumer Economics, University of Illinois, Champaign-Urbana; Roland L. Weinsier, M.D. Ph.D., C. E. Butterworth Jr. Professor and Chair, Department of Nutritional Sciences, University of Alabama in Birmingham; Lisa Young, M.S., R.D., Adjunct Professor, Department of Nutrition and Food Studies, New York University, New York.

To the degree that we are successful in achieving our goals for *Volumetrics*—bringing to the public a new science-based approach to weight management that is both enjoyable and healthful—we are indebted to everyone listed here, and many others who have helped us in ways large and small. To the degree that we fall short, the fault is ours alone.

Part 1:

What Is Volumetrics?

Introduction

WELCOME TO *The Volumetrics Weight-Control Plan,* the first book to use breakthrough new research on the science of satiety to help you control your eating habits. What is satiety? It's the feeling of fullness at the end of a meal, the feeling that you are no longer hungry. The more satiety you feel after a meal, the less you'll eat at the next one.

Satiety is the missing ingredient in weight management. Cut calories by simply eating less, and you'll feel hungry and deprived. You may be able to stick to such a diet for the short term, but to become successful at lifelong weight management, you'll need an eating pattern that lets you feel full with fewer calories.

The primary way to do this is to get smart about your food choices. For any given level of calories, some foods will have a small effect on satiety, others a large one. The right food choices will help you control hunger *and* eat fewer calories, so you can lose weight, keep it off, and stay healthy.

There's no secret to weight management: Consume fewer calories and burn more in physical activity. You can't lose weight without controlling calories. But you *can* control calories without feeling hungry. Feeling full and satisfied while eating foods you like is a critical component of our approach to weight management.

The basic strategy of Volumetrics *is to eat a satisfying volume of food while controlling calories and meeting nutrient requirements.*

THE FOODS YOU CHOOSE

Which foods should you choose?

Surprisingly, foods with a high water content have a big impact on satiety. But you can't simply drink lots of water, which quenches thirst without sating hunger. You'll need to eat more *foods* that are naturally rich in water, such as fruits, vegetables, low-fat milk, and cooked grains, as well as lean meats, poultry, fish, and beans. It also means eating more water-rich dishes: soups, stews, casseroles, pasta with vegetables, and fruit-based desserts. On the other hand, you'll have to be very careful about foods that are very low in water: high-fat foods like potato chips, but also low-fat and fat-free foods that contain very little moisture, like pretzels, crackers, and fat-free cookies.

Why is water so helpful in controlling calories? It dilutes the calories in a given amount of food. When you add water-rich blueberries to your breakfast cereal, or water-rich eggplant to your lasagna, you add food volume but few calories. *You can eat more for the same calories.* This property of foods—the calories in a given portion—is the core concept of this book. We call it by its scientific term, *energy density.*

Water is only one of many food elements that affect satiety and energy density. In addition to water, fiber can be added to foods to lower the calories in a portion. It provides bulk without a lot of calories. So by strategically increasing the water and fiber content of meals—with the addition of fruits, vegetables, and whole grains you can dramatically cut the calories per portion—you lower the energy density. On the other hand, the component of foods that increases the energy density the most is fat. Fat has more than twice as many calories per portion as either carbohydrate or protein. So if you cut fat, you can lower the energy density of a meal. You can combine these strategies: Increase the water and fiber content of foods while lowering the fat content to get satisfying portions with few calories.

This book is based on recent research showing how foods affect hunger and satiety, which in turn has led to new ways to manage weight. Each of the major elements that makes up food—fat, carbohydrates, protein, water—has an effect on satiety. So do other dietary components: sugar, fiber, alcohol, and sugar and fat substitutes. In the next part of the book, we explore these influences in detail so you can learn the basic principles of choosing a lower-calorie, more satisfying diet.

If you've suffered through dietary deprivation to lose weight, you may find it hard to believe that you can eat more food, feel full, and still reduce your total caloric intake. To make our program work, some people, if they choose lots of foods that have only few calories in a portion, may actually have to retrain themselves to eat *larger* portions than they do now.

We won't ask you to greatly restrict your food choices. You won't have to cut out all the fat from your diet, live on rabbit food, subsist on foods on a "free" list, or avoid any food. *Volumetrics* allows a wide choice of foods. You'll be able to eat bread, pasta, rice, beef, chicken, fish and seafood, dairy products, vegetables, and fruits.

To do so while cutting calories, we'll show you how to make changes such as adding vegetables to a risotto, or choosing fruit over fat-free cookies for dessert. You'll also gain greater understanding of the kinds of foods that are deceptively easy to overeat, whether it's cheese, chocolate, raisins, or pretzels. We won't ask you to ban them. That's not our style, because it's not a style that works. Instead, we will give you specific strategies so you can enjoy them without taking in too many calories. *Volumetrics* is not really a diet at all, but a new way to choose satisfying, lower-calorie foods.

While we emphasize lowering the energy density of your dietary pattern because that's the best way to eat a satisfying amount of food, we don't want you to get the impression that energy-dense foods are "bad" or "forbidden." Who wants to go through life without chocolate? Favorite foods, even if they are high in energy density, have a place in your dietary pattern. But you will have to *plan* for them. If you rely on the body's satiety signals to stop you eating chocolate, you'll consume too many calories. So you'll need to satisfy your hunger with foods of lower energy density, and then enjoy high-energy-dense foods in appropriate portions. If the meal itself is satiating, a half-ounce of chocolate is a satisfying ending.

Our nondieting approach extends to the weight loss program, which emphasizes only a modest caloric "deficit," rather than a large one that results in quick weight loss. You may lose weight more gradually than on other weight loss programs, but you won't feel deprived.

Because we emphasize foods with plenty of volume for their calories, we call our book *The Volumetrics Weight-Control Plan*. We're interested in both the volume and the weight of food you can eat since both affect satiety. If you follow our suggestions, your plate will be full of food and you will feel full. By making it easier to cut calories, this approach makes it easier to reduce the volume that's most troublesome: your own.

WHAT'S INCLUDED IN *VOLUMETRICS*

The Volumetrics Weight-Control Plan is divided into seven sections:

Part 1: What Is *Volumetrics*? In the introduction, we discuss the main themes of this book. In the next chapter, "The Energy Density Breakthrough," we'll explain the scientific breakthrough that indicates that eating a satisfying volume of food is critical for managing hunger while reducing calories.

Part 2: How to Lose Weight and Keep It Off. Here is the latest research on how to plan a program to lose weight, improve your health, and increase your chances of keeping the weight off.

Part 3: What We Eat and Drink. In this section, we'll tell you what the scientific evidence shows us about how fat, carbohydrates (including sugar), protein, alcohol, and water and other beverages affect how much you eat and how full you feel. The chapter "Soup" is a case study that illustrates how a low-calorie, high-volume food promotes satiety with few calories.

Part 4: The Food Guide. What are the best foods to choose to make your dietary pattern more *Volumetric*? Here's a detailed list of over 600 foods, divided into four categories, to help you select a satisfying, lower-calorie diet. You can see at a glance how to make more satisfying food choices in each food group. In this section, we'll also show you how to use our principles to choose a well-balanced, nutritionally adequate diet consistent with the USDA's Food Guide Pyramid.

Part 5: The Menu Plan. Ready? Our menu plans won't feel like a conventional diet: The calories are low enough to provide weight loss but not so low that you'll feel deprived. The volume of food you can eat is bigger, and the choices are wider than in a traditional weight loss program. In this section, we provide calorie-controlled menus for breakfast, lunch, dinner, and snacks (including desserts). You can mix and match menus to design a personal weight loss eating plan at either 1,600 or 2,000 calories. We also give you tips on how to adjust the plan to other calorie levels. Many of the menus take advantage of our more than fifty delicious, easy-to-prepare recipes. This section also includes step-by-step demonstrations of how to modify favorite recipes.

Part 6: An Active Life. Becoming more physically active will help you burn more calories, increase metabolism, and stay committed to a healthier way of eating. You don't have to become an athlete to keep the weight off. Here's a program that's easy to fit into a busy life.

Part 7: The Satiety Lifestyle. Hunger and satiety are affected by more than the type of foods you eat. How many calories you eat is influenced by how big a package you buy in the supermarket, how many different foods you pile onto your plate, and whether you're watching television while you eat. In this section, we explore the many environmental influences on eating and give you ways to manage them.

ARE YOU PREPARED FOR A NEW WEIGHT MANAGEMENT PATH?

You can use this book to lose weight. We've designed it that way. But the power of *Volumetrics* goes beyond short-term weight loss to long-term weight management. *It's a lifestyle plan, not a diet.* Any program that gets you to consume fewer calories in the short term will help you lose weight. The hardest part is keeping the weight from returning, and preventing the seemingly inevitable, slow weight gain that occurs with the years. That's where this book will be most helpful.

While we believe this new approach is a fundamental breakthrough in weight management, we know it won't solve every eating problem; in particular, if your overeating is rooted in depression or has other emotional causes, you will need to address these issues, perhaps with a therapist, before you are ready to adopt the eating style in this book. On the other hand, if you are under medical treatment for obesity (or for a medical condition like high blood pressure that is affected by body weight), this book may be particularly useful to you, but do show it to your health care provider first.

Volumetrics is primarily about the foods you eat. If you've endured a series of weight loss diets over the years, with their long lists of foods to avoid—and the attendant feelings of hunger and deprivation, not to mention symptoms such as fatigue and difficulty concentrating—our positive *Volumetrics* approach will be a welcome change. It's a sound program, based on the latest nutritional guidelines that have been carefully developed to ensure enough essential nutrients while lowering the risk of chronic disease. We'll help you avoid dieting traps that make life difficult without really helping you lose weight and keep it off.

While we can make losing weight and keeping it off easier, we can't make it effortless. Both authors of this book know from personal experience that changing the way you eat is not a simple affair. It takes skill and planning and knowledge and dedication. *Volumetrics* offers the tools to make those changes, to manage hunger and appetite so that you can feel satisfied without overeating. If you're already committed to change—if you've made some changes in how you eat, but are eager to learn new ones that will help you in the lifelong challenge of weight management—you'll find *Volumetrics* an invaluable ally. It will allow you to eat healthfully, enjoy your favorite foods in satisfying portions, feel full, and control calories.

The Principles of Volumetrics

What's the ideal weight loss program? It's one that satisfies hunger, reduces calories, meets nutritional needs and includes physical activity. It must be enjoyable, and thus, sustainable.

Here is the foundation of our plan. You'll learn the details as you read *Volumetrics*.

Element	Recommendation	Comments
Energy (Calories)	Reduce usual intake by 500–1000 calories/day, depending on your weight-loss goal.	Should lead to weight loss of 1 to 2 lb/week.
Fat	20% to 30% of total calories.	Look for foods reduced in both fat and energy density.
Carbohydrates	55% or more of total calories.	Emphasize carbohydrates from whole grains, vegetables and fruits. These are more satiating.
Fiber	20 to 30 grams/day.	Choose not only whole grains, but fiber-rich breakfast cereals, and whole fruits and vegetables more often than juices. Fiber modestly lowers energy density, and it also increases satiety.
Sugars	Choose a diet moderate in added sugars.	Lower intake of sugary drinks, which add calories with little satiety. Use modest amounts of sugar to make nutritious foods of low energy density more palatable.
Protein	Maintain intake at 0.4 grams per pound body weight, approximately 15% of total calories.	More satiating than carbohydrate or fat. During weight loss, adequate amounts needed to prevent muscle loss and thus maintain metabolic rate. Make low-energy-dense choices such as beans, low-fat fish, poultry without skin and lean meats.

Alcohol	Limit to one drink/day for women, 2 drinks/day for men.	Consume with meals of low-fat, low-energy-dense foods. Limit evening drinking and snacking.
Water	For optimal health, consume about 9 cups/day for women, 12 cups/day for men. Can come from water in foods or beverages.	Replace sugary drinks with water. Consume more foods with high-water content, which will also increase satiety.
Physical Activity	At least 30 minutes or more of moderate-intensity physical activity on most, and preferably all, days of the week. Include resistance training twice a week.	Brisk walking at 3 to 4 m.p.h is ideal for most people, but anything that gets you moving is good. Include some activities of longer duration for better fat burning. Also, reduce sedentary time with lifestyle activities such as gardening.

The Energy Density Breakthrough

To eat is a necessity, but to eat intelligently is an art.
—La Rochefoucauld, *Maxims*, 1665

HOW CAN YOU EAT SATISFYING PORTIONS of food and still take in fewer calories? How can certain food choices lead to extra calories and weight gain while others make it easy to feel full while you lose weight? The answer lies in the implications of an observation so simple that, until now, it's been nearly invisible, even to scientists who study eating behavior:

Over the course of a day or two, a person eats about the same weight of food.

It varies by individual, of course. You don't eat the same amount as your friends, but on average the weight of food you ate on a daily basis last week will probably be quite similar to the weight of food you eat this week.

Therefore, if you maintain the usual amount of food you eat, yet lower the calories in each portion, you'll consume fewer calories and feel just as full.

Let's consider what this means for a typical meal.

A NIGHT OUT

It's Friday night, and you and your friends or family are eating out at your favorite Chinese restaurant. You order a stir-fry with steak and vegetables in the chef's special sauce, served over rice. How many calories are you consuming? That depends on your chef. If he has a heavy hand with the oil, the calories might shoot up; on the other hand, if he has increased the amount of water or vegetables in his special sauce, calories will decrease. But you won't know all that when you ladle a spoonful of stir-fry over your rice.

If you're used to eating a cup of stir-fry over a cup of rice, you'll likely eat that much, even if the calories in the cup are twice—or half—what they usually are.

Why do people eat a constant weight of food? It may seem a strange eating strategy, but it really isn't. When you serve yourself a portion of food, in most cases you don't know how many calories are in it. You are faced with situations like this all the time, and what you are likely to do, and what it makes sense to do, is to rely on your previous experience with that type of food. You choose a portion of the food that you have learned is appropriate to leave you satisfied, even if there are big differences in the calories in a portion.

The surprising thing is that a lower-calorie portion of food will satisfy you as much as a higher-calorie portion. Let's see what a big difference this approach makes in how much you can eat.

A HANDFUL OF FOOD—OR A BOWLFUL?

It's Saturday afternoon and you want a little snack. You want to keep it under 100 calories. There are fresh grapes in the refrigerator and raisins in the pantry. Both are healthy snacks; in fact, they are the same food! Raisins, after all, are simply dried grapes. If you choose raisins, however, you'll be able to consume only ¼ cup rather than 1⅔ cups of grapes for your 100 calories:

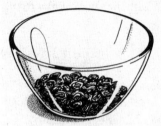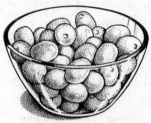

For 100 calories, you can eat ¼ cup of raisins—or nearly 2 cups of grapes.

Which is likely to fill you up more?

A TOMATO LESSON

Let's take another example. It's summer, and you've just bought—or picked—a fresh garden tomato, so red and juicy that you can't wait to get it back to your kitchen to slice and eat it. Your pantry also holds fat-free pretzels. Which is a more filling snack?

You probably guessed by now that it's tomatoes. But do you know how much more you can eat? If you eat an entire medium tomato, you'll take in 25 calories. To keep your pretzels down to that calorie level, though, you'll be able to eat only ¼ ounce—about 4 or 5 tiny sticks. Ounce for ounce, pretzels have about twenty times as many calories as tomatoes!

We're not suggesting that you snack only on tomatoes. This is a crucial point. Previous weight management books have recommended diets that tell you to cut back on every gram of fat—to forget about meat, to drop sweets. We won't tell you to do that. Rather, we'll give you basic information so you can make smart choices in what you eat.

For example, if you snack on pretzels, with more than 100 calories in each ounce, you may take in several hundred calories before your body tells you that it's full. But you don't need to skip the pretzels. Perhaps you'll want to eat the sliced tomato drizzled with a little balsamic vinegar and fresh black pepper and salt, *and* an ounce of pretzels—you'll consume only 125 calories. Even if you drizzle a teaspoon of olive oil over your tomato, and eat it with the pretzels, your total is still only 165 calories. You'll have eaten a satisfying portion and will feel fuller than with the same calories from pretzels alone.

ENERGY DENSITY

If you are trying to consume fewer calories, what is critical is the amount of calories in a given portion of food. A food that is of high energy density provides a large amount of calories in a small weight, while a food of low energy density has fewer calories for the same weight. With foods of lower energy density, you can eat a larger portion for the same calories.

Fat is the most energy dense element of food at 9 calories per gram, alcohol is next at 7, followed by protein and carbohydrates each at 4, and water at 0:

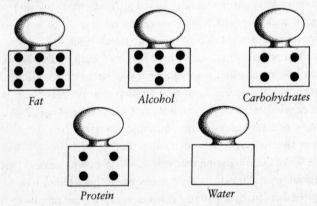

Fat   Alcohol   Carbohydrates

Protein   Water

Each of these scale weights is one gram, but the calories, represented by dots, vary enormously. Water has none, carbohydrates and protein each have four, but fat crams nine calories (dots) in each gram, making it the most energy-dense of nutrients.

It's the mix of these elements that determines the energy density of a food. Substitute carbohydrate for fat, and you lower a food's energy density. Increasing the water content of a food is even more effective. Remember the grapes versus raisins illustration above? The only difference between the two foods is their water content.

Low-water foods, even those that are virtually fat-free, can be as energy dense as high-fat foods. Compare cheddar cheese and a classic "diet" food: Melba toast. Everyone knows that cheddar cheese can be a problem food for the calorie-conscious. It's high in fat. But these fat calories are diluted by the water and protein in cheese so that its energy density is 4 calories per gram. Three ounces of cheddar cheese has nearly 350 calories.

But Melba toast *also* has an energy density of 4 calories per gram. With little or no water, there is nothing to dilute the pure carbohydrate's energy density. Eating 3 ounces of Melba toast also provides 350 calories. So if you eat the same size portion, you'll consume as many calories from fat-free, high-carbohydrate snacks as from high-fat foods of similar energy density.

You can see the interplay between fat and water even more clearly if you compare a chocolate bar to a glass of chocolate whole milk. Both are high in fat, but the chocolate milk contains much more water. So, a 1½-ounce milk chocolate bar has 230 calories, while an 8-ounce glass of chocolate milk made with whole milk has 250 calories. For about the same calories, you get a portion that is five times bigger than the chocolate bar. The water in the milk lowered the energy density. You could lower the energy density even more if you also lowered the fat content. If you chose chocolate milk made with low-fat (1 percent) milk, in 8 ounces you would take in only 158 calories. Fat matters for energy density, but water matters more. When we increased the water content, you could have five times more; when we reduced the fat content, you could have about one and a half times more. Water can be added to foods to provide a more satisfying portion and it can lower the energy density of any food, even those high in fat.

The study of energy density has opened up a new array of weight control strategies. Sure, it's important to moderate your fat intake since it packs so many calories into a portion. But it's only part of the story. It's also important to eat more foods that have a high water content, including cooked grains, vegetables, fruits, soups, and stews. Sometimes, lowering the energy density of a family recipe is as simple as adding naturally water-rich vegetables. When you do this, you can eat more for the same number of calories, or you can eat your usual portion and take in fewer calories. It's a positive approach, certainly a lot more fun than trying to squeeze the fat out of every food you put in your mouth. In the next section, we'll illustrate how easy this new approach can be.

How to Calculate Energy Density

Let us introduce a single number that is so important that it should be added to every food that carries a nutrition label: *calories per gram*. It's a measure of energy density. Here's how to calculate it:

$$\frac{\text{Calories}}{\text{Gram}} = \text{Energy density (abbreviated E.D.)}$$

A *calorie* is a measure of the amount of heat produced by metabolizing food. This heat provides the *energy* that powers your body.

A *gram* is a measure of weight (there are about 28 grams in an ounce).

So calories per gram measures how much energy you'll get from a given weight of food. If one food has an energy density of 1.0, while another has an energy density of 2.0, you'll get twice as many calories from the same size serving of the second food.

While the "Nutrition Facts" label on foods doesn't yet include energy density, you can easily calculate it from two facts that *are* there: calories and weight in grams. You can find this information on the top of the label, as we illustrate below. We'll use as our example a low-fat frozen yogurt:

Serving size. This tells you the standard serving size of the food, and, in parentheses, the weight in grams. For this frozen yogurt, that's 98 grams.

Calories. Here, it's 160.

Nutrition Facts
Serving Size 1/2 cup (98g)
Servings Per Container 4

Amount Per Serving

Calories 160 Calories from Fat 25

Now comes the fun part: To calculate the energy density, divide the calories by the weight: 160 divided by 98 yields 1.6. Even if you don't have a calculator and aren't good at math in your head, you can get a pretty good idea of a food's energy density by comparing calories to grams. If the calories are less than the grams, that food has an energy density below 1.0. If calories are twice the grams (e.g., 200 calories, 100 grams), that food has an energy density of 2.0. And so forth. Use this quick method to compare similar foods when you're shopping. We also give you a list of the energy densities of over 600 foods in "The Food Guide" (p. 105).

We have divided foods into the following four categories:

Category 1: Very Low-Energy-Dense Foods. E.D. less than 0.6: Includes most fruits and vegetables, skim milk, and broth-based soups.

Category 2: Low-Energy-Dense Foods. E.D. 0.6 to 1.5: Includes many cooked grains, breakfast cereals with low-fat milk, low-fat meats, beans and legumes, low-fat mixed dishes, and salads.

Category 3: Medium-Energy-Dense Foods. E.D. 1.5 to 4.0: Includes meats, cheeses, high-fat mixed dishes, salad dressings, some snack foods.

Category 4: High-Energy-Dense Foods. E.D. 4.0 to 9.0: Includes crackers, chips, chocolate candies, cookies, nuts, butter, and full-fat condiments.

MORE FOOD, PLEASE

Here are two portions of an Italian pasta salad that provide 200 calories:

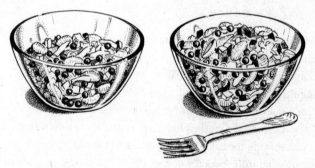

Italian Pasta Salad: With less pasta and more vegetables,
the 200 calorie serving on the right gives you nearly twice as much to eat.

If you think the serving on the right looks bigger, you're right. It is. It's about 2 cups of food, compared to 1⅓ cups of food for the salad on the left. Yet both provide 200 calories. The difference isn't the fat. Both are low-fat dishes, with about 18 percent of calories from fat. Each portion is made with 2 tablespoons part-skim mozzarella, about 1 tablespoon low-calorie Italian dressing, and 1 tablespoon lean diced ham per serving.

The difference is the ratio of pasta to vegetables. There is slightly less pasta in the portion on the right: ½ rather than ¾ cup. But the amount of vegetables is much greater in the one on the right: ⅓ cup of carrots versus a skimpy 1½ tablespoons, ⅓ cup each of sliced zucchini and diced tomatoes versus 1 tablespoon each in the one on the left.

Modest differences, but they add up to a portion of food that's nearly double for the same calories. The energy density goes down from a modest 1.2 calories per gram to a low 0.8 calories per gram (see "How to Calculate Energy Density, p. 14). This means that if you ate the same 3-ounce portion, you would take in about 100 calories from the higher-energy-dense salad and about 70 from the lower-energy-dense salad.

But how do we know that people won't just eat more of the pasta salad on the right? Good question. Let us show you how scientists have come to appreciate the impact of energy density on caloric intake and weight management.

THE BREAKTHROUGH

Many diets emphasize the importance of a particular nutrient for weight control. A few years ago people were convinced that it was fat that was making them fat. With the focus on fat, the importance of the effects of energy density on food intake and satiety was not appreciated. Often high-fat foods are high in energy density, and it was assumed that the effects of fat and energy density on food intake were the same. But if you recall the examples we gave earlier of what influences the energy density of foods, we showed you that the water content of foods can have an even bigger effect on energy density than fat. So we can separate the effects of fat and energy density by varying the water content of foods. When we do

Pumping Up Your Food

Energy density is the ratio of calories to the *weight* of food. In general, portions that weigh more are also bigger in volume. But what about pure *volume*? What about air? Is food that's puffed up with air more satisfying than a smaller, packed-down portion?

The answer is yes. The volume of food really does affect how satisfied you feel and how much you eat. We showed this by simply adding air to strawberry smoothies. We took exactly the same ingredients and put them in the blender for different amounts of time so that we ended up with drinks that were a half, three-quarters, or a full glass. Then we gave them to young men to drink a half-hour before lunch. The bigger the smoothie, the less they ate at lunch: 12 percent less following the biggest drink compared to the smallest. They also felt fuller after the bigger drink, and they didn't make up the calories later in the day.

We're not suggesting you try to fill up on lots of airy foods. You might get a stomach ache, and would probably burp a lot! But this study does show that you can trick your senses into believing you have eaten more food by pumping up the volume. You see a bigger portion, and you get more sensory stimulation as you consume it.

Try whipped foods in moderation such as low-fat frozen desserts. Get creative with blender drinks. Choose air-popped popcorn; its energy density is not low, but it takes 3 cups to give you 90 calories (try it without butter—add low-fat seasoning instead). Foods with irregular shapes also produce a bigger volume in a given portion because they don't pack down. Think of flaky or puffed cereals.

In other words: Think big!

---

this, we see that it is the energy density of foods that affects satiety and how much is eaten.

Consider these findings:

- Studies in the Netherlands, Britain, and the United States have shown that when energy density of the diet was held constant, no matter what the fat content, people ate the same weight of food daily. This meant that daily calorie intake was also the same. These studies demonstrate that the energy density, not the fat content of diets, affects how many calories are eaten.

- In a U.S. survey looking at people's usual intakes, when people were asked to weigh the foods they ate for 4 days, it was confirmed that on average people ate the same weight of food each day. This again suggests that it is the energy density of the diet that determines daily calorie intake.

- Obese people have more energy-dense dietary patterns than normal-weight individuals. In one survey, very obese men and women in the United States not only ate lots of energy-dense foods (big portions of meats, full-fat milk and cheese, fried eggs, high-fat desserts), but also very few low-energy-dense foods (salads, fruit, skim milk). Dutch researchers found that lean people have diets of lower energy density than obese people. The message is clear: Eating a high-energy-dense diet is associated with elevated body weight.

What matters to *you*, though, is what happens when you lower the energy density of your customary meals. Will you spontaneously consume fewer calories? To find out, come to our "Eating Lab."

THE PASTA EXPERIMENTS

Here at the Laboratory for the Study of Human Ingestive Behavior at Penn State, the atmosphere may not be romantic, but the food is good. It has to be. We need to make sure that all the foods we serve are equally tasty, so we can measure other influences on how much people eat. That's what graduate student Elizabeth Bell did when she served normal-weight women breakfast, lunch, dinner, and snacks over three 2-day periods. At meals, they could eat as much of a main dish as they wanted.

The main dishes were all low in fat, but they varied in energy density. For example, for lunch the women were served a pasta dish (similar to the Italian pasta salad illustrated on p. 15). On some days, the pasta salad had fewer vegetables and more pasta, so it had more calories in each portion; on others, we replaced some of the pasta with extra chopped vegetables, so it had fewer calories in each portion. Whether we served them high-, medium-, or low-energy-density main dishes, each woman ate the same amount of food, about 3 pounds total for each day. As a result, on the low-energy-density days, they consumed 30 percent fewer calories than on the high-energy-density days.

They felt just as full and satisfied.

But they were consuming about 400 fewer calories each day.

YOU DON'T HAVE TO CHANGE YOUR ENTIRE DIET

Too often, when a new weight management idea becomes popular, people take it too far.

This could happen if you choose only foods of *very* low energy density, attempting to subsist on, for instance, carrots, tomatoes, and chicken rice soup. Don't! Extremes backfire. Forbid a food and you may crave it. Such diets are also unhealthy.

The good news is that it's not necessary. You don't need to change everything you eat, or to give up your favorite foods. We showed this in a study in which we asked people to change only *half* the foods they ate every day. For 4 days at a time, lean and over-weight women ate all their meals in the Eating Lab. We required them to eat the entire portion of main dishes that supplied half the calories they normally ate at each meal, and then let them eat what-ever they wanted from a wide selection of foods. For example, for dinner one day we served chicken-rice Florentine as a main dish, and in addition the women could eat as much plain chicken breast, pota-toes, broccoli and cauliflower, salad, rolls and butter, and dessert as they wanted. They could also eat whatever they liked between meals.

When we lowered the energy density of the required main dishes, the women ate fewer total calories over each day. What was particu-larly exciting was that they didn't consume any more of the "free" foods we offered them at each meal, or that they chose on their own as snacks. The women were not consciously dieting, yet when they ate the low-energy-dense meals, they consumed 16 percent fewer calories over the 4 days of the study, and reported feeling just as full.

What we really like about this study is that it points the way to a sensible strategy to control calories: Eat some filling low-

How Do Volumetric Foods Fill You Up on Fewer Calories?

It seems too simple. How can eating foods of low energy density fill you up on fewer calories? The answer is that your body has many "satiety" systems that signal that you've eaten enough, and high-volume foods activate most of them. Let's consider what happens when you sit down to a *Volumetric* meal. Here's how it affects satiety:

Mind. You've grown up with ideas about appropriate portions of food to satisfy hunger. Being able to select a normal portion of food, even as you limit calories, fits into your expectations that the meal will be satisfying.

Eyes. A meal begins with the eyes. When you see a big, appetizing plate of food in front of you, that increases your expectation that you'll feel satiated at the end of the meal.

Nose and mouth. As you smell, chew, taste, and swallow the food, you get sensory pleasure. With a bigger volume of food, there's more food to eat, so these taste and other sensory satiety signals that travel to your brain last longer.

Stomach. A bigger volume of food fills your stomach, activating "stretch" receptors. These stretch receptors tell the brain that a satisfying amount of food has been eaten. As it fills, the stomach contracts rhythmically, breaking food into tiny particles that can pass into the intestines. These rhythmic contractions are part of satiety, and they are similar whether breaking down a pound of food that has 500 calories or a pound that has 1,500 calories. A larger portion of food also takes longer to travel through the stomach than a smaller portion, prolonging satiety signals.

Liver, pancreas, small intestine, large intestine. As the food travels through the gut, a series of satiety signals continues to be sent to the brain. The small intestine, for example, releases cholecystokinin (CCK), dubbed the "satiety hormone." A large volume of food stimulates more of these satiety signals as it moves through the digestive system.

Eating a normal portion of food is needed for these systems to work properly. Eating in a healthful *Volumetrics* dietary pattern is the first step to controlling calories without feeling hungry.

energy-dense, *Volumetric* foods at most meals, so you can still enjoy small portions of foods higher in energy density. By eating more foods low in energy density you'll be consuming a satisfying volume of food that controls hunger and leaves you feeling full on fewer calories. But you won't have to give up any particular food. You won't feel like you are on a "diet."

CAN THIS REALLY HELP ME LOSE WEIGHT?

The research on energy density, eating, and weight is new. Long-term weight management clinical trials have not yet been conducted, although they are in the works. There has, however, been one study looking at the effects of energy density on food intake and body weight over 14 days. Six normal-weight men took all of their meals at a lab in Scotland during three fourteen-day test periods during which the energy density varied. The higher the energy density, the higher the daily calorie intake. Over the two weeks during which the men ate the diet that was highest in energy density, they gained about two pounds; on the lowest energy-dense diet over two weeks, they lost about two pounds. In addition, a look at successful university-based and commercial weight management programs reveals that lowering energy density plays a crucial strategic role.

In Alabama, one program has been helping people lose weight using the principles of *Volumetrics* for 25 years. In 1976, Roland L. Weinsier of the University of Alabama at Birmingham began a weight-loss program that helped people eat substantially fewer calories by switching from a high-fat, energy-dense diet to one that was lower in fat and energy density. In 1983, he showed that people who stayed on a low-energy-dense weight loss plan maintained the lost weight, and 80 percent were at their new lower body weight or below 2 years later. "The program is effective in people who are mildly overweight—or massively obese," says Weinsier. "It works in men and women." The program includes weekly sessions that teach a lifestyle of low-energy-density eating and increased physical activity. "We preach the importance of eating large amounts of food. That's counterintuitive. But the volume of food becomes large enough that for many people the food they have to eat is more than they ate when they were gaining weight."

Teaching people how to eat more satisfying, lower-calorie meals is also central to other weight management programs. While Weight Watchers' "1, 2, 3" program lets people choose any foods they want for their calorie level, explains lead scientist Karen Miller-Kovachs, "people quickly learn that grains, fruits, and vegetables leave them full at the end of the day, but that chocolate and cheesecake leave them hungry." Says Duke University Diet & Fitness Centers' nutrition director Terry Brownlee, "We combine really low-energy-dense foods, like big salads and fruit portions, with foods higher in energy density that have some fat for taste, like hamburgers or steak. For example, we do a taco salad—a bed of nice greens, a few baked chips, a little sprinkle of cheese, a couple of olives, and lean ground beef mixed with barley. I often hear, 'I'm really surprised at how satisfied I feel.'"

VOLUMETRICS

By now, you're probably eager to learn how to integrate these principles into your own weight management plan. In Part 3 (p. 39), we'll explore in more detail just how different nutritional factors, such as fat and fiber and protein and water, affect energy density and satiety. We'll help you understand not just which foods are loaded with calories, but what kinds of foods, eaten under which circumstances, allow you to consume fewer calories and still be satisfied. And we'll point out the hidden calorie traps, the seemingly innocuous foods that can sneak in unwanted calories without your body recognizing them.

We can't guarantee that you'll lose weight and keep it off. To lose weight, you'll have to take in fewer calories than you burn; to keep it off, you'll have to take in the same number of calories as you burn. But we can show you how to consume fewer calories while enjoying a satisfying portion of food.

SUMMARY

- If you maintain the usual volume of food you eat, yet lower the calories in each portion, you'll consume fewer calories and feel just as full.

- Foods can vary enormously in energy density. For the same calories, you can eat ¼ cup raisins, or 1⅔ cups of grapes. For the same calories, you can eat twenty times as much tomato by weight as pretzels!

- A high-fat diet promotes weight gain because it's high in energy density. Just cutting fat won't help you lose weight, unless you also limit low-fat or fat-free foods that are high in energy density.

- Water that's incorporated into food plays a crucial role in controlling hunger. To lower the energy density of your diet, eat more foods that are high in water, including cooked grains, fruits, vegetables, soups, and stews.

- You don't have to change your entire diet. By eating more meals and snacks that are lower in energy density, you can still enjoy reasonable portions of your favorite energy-dense foods while controlling calories.

- Lowering your diet's overall energy density, as part of an integrated program of exercise and behavioral management, can result in significant weight loss that is sustained over time.

Part 2:

How to Lose Weight and Keep It Off

THE PRINCIPLES OF *VOLUMETRICS* are designed to help everyone eat a more satisfying diet while controlling calories. If you're at a healthy weight now, employ these principles to prevent weight gain. You can use the tips to make better food choices, and cook the recipes that come later, without engaging in a formal plan.

If you need or want to lose weight, on the other hand, you'll need a more deliberate weight management plan. It's too hard to go on a weight loss diet just to see the weight return a few months later. Fortunately, the science of weight management has advanced significantly in the last few years. In this section, we'll show you how to plan a weight loss program, including how to determine how much weight you'll need to lose, how fast to lose it, and how many calories to cut on a daily basis to achieve that. We'll help you understand how weight management can improve your health, and how to keep the weight off.

Creating Your Own Weight Management Program

AT THE UNIVERSITY OF PENNSYLVANIA in Philadelphia, sixty obese women (average weight: 218 pounds) participated in a 48-week weight loss clinic program. They were asked, "How much weight do you want to lose?" Each woman described a "dream weight," "happy weight," "acceptable weight," and "disappointed weight." "Dream" weight meant losing an average of 70 pounds (32 percent of body weight), while "disappointed" weight loss was 37 pounds. In the end, the actual weight loss was 35 pounds, even below "disappointed" weight.

Yet the doctors running the program were pleased. The women may not have been happy, but they were healthier. After all, they had lost 16 percent of their body weight, substantially lowering their risk of heart disease, stroke, diabetes, and other risk factors associated with obesity. If you're overweight or obese, losing as little as 5–10 percent of your body weight can improve health.

What are *your* expectations for weight loss? It's the first place to start in planning a weight loss program. If you expect too much—if you want a "dream body"—you may wind up feeling like a failure, even as you achieve success. If you do achieve your dream weight through a lifestyle you can't sustain, you may simply regain much of the weight. On the other hand, if you choose a reasonable weight loss goal, and follow a sensible program of *Volumetric* eating and increased physical activity, you *can* lose a significant amount of weight—and keep it off.

This is very good news. Just a few years ago, weight management experts weren't sure how successful weight management was in the long term. They knew people could lose weight, but could they keep it off? Now there's a solid scientific basis for optimism.

The National Weight Loss Registry, for example, is a national survey of over 2,500 men and women who've lost over 30 pounds and kept it off at least a year (average weight loss: 66 pounds). "We've learned that successful weight loss and maintenance is possible," says researcher Mary Lou Klem of the University of Pittsburgh School of Medicine, where the registry is coordinated. "People overwhelmingly tell us that they use both diet and exercise to lose the weight and keep it off. They report really positive changes in the quality of life."

In the last few years, weight management experts have determined that a well-designed diet-and-exercise program can greatly improve your odds of weight management success. The National Institutes of Health (NIH) recently published science-based weight management guidelines. They call it "the evidence report," because they've culled the scientific literature for methods that are proven to work. In this chapter, we'll share those methods.

DO YOU NEED TO LOSE WEIGHT FOR HEALTH?

If you are reading this book, chances are you already believe that losing weight or avoiding weight gain is a healthy choice. You may already know of the health risks linked to being overweight or obese: high blood pressure, high blood cholesterol levels, type 2 diabetes, heart disease, stroke, gallbladder disease, osteoarthritis, sleep apnea and respiratory problems, and a slight increase in risk of developing certain cancers (breast, prostate, colon). Obesity is an independent factor in raising these health risks, which increase your chances of dying prematurely. Lose weight, and your health risks go down, quickly. (If you have a family history of heart disease—a father or uncle who had a heart attack before age 55, a mother or aunt before age 65—lowering your cardiovascular health risks by managing your weight is even more critical. If you smoke, which also increases the health risks of obesity, the first step is to quit smoking, then use the principles of this book to lose weight.)

To figure out whether you need to lose weight to become healthier, you'll need to determine whether you are "overweight" or "obese." Both refer to a condition of too much body fat. Scientists gauge body fat by a special ratio of weight-to-height called the Body Mass Index (BMI), which accurately reflects body fat in the vast majority of adult men and women. The main exceptions are people who are very fit and muscular, whose greater weight is due to having more muscle, not fat. To figure out your current BMI you can get a rough estimate from our chart "What's Your BMI?" (p. 29) or find your calculator:

1   Multiply your height in inches by itself. For example, if you are 5'8", that's 68 inches, and 68 times 68 equals 4,624.

2   Now divide your weight in pounds by that number. Thus, if you weigh 164 pounds, you'd divide 164 by 4,624, and get 0.03546.

3   Finally, multiply that number by 704.5. This is your BMI; in this case, 25.

Here's how to interpret it:

- **BMI under 18.5.** You are underweight, which is associated with health risks. Dieting would be dangerous to your health. Work on eating a nutritious diet and becoming more fit.

- **BMI of 18.5 to 25.** You are normal weight. Eat a nutritious diet, stay fit, and maintain your weight.

- **BMI of 25 to 30.** You are overweight. For a BMI of 25 to 27, the increase in health risk is modest, but strive to prevent further weight gain. Health risks begin to rise significantly with a BMI over 27. If your BMI is 27–30, begin a weight loss program.

- **BMI of 30 to 35.** You are obese. Your health risks are greatly increased. Lose weight now, especially through a sensible diet and increased exercise, and you will markedly reduce your health risk factors such as high blood pressure or high cholesterol. If you do have these or other risk factors, see your physician about planning a weight loss plan; bring this book.

- **BMI over 35.** You are severely obese. See your physician about losing weight; bring this book.

At any given weight, you are at increased risk of heart disease and diabetes if you carry your weight around the middle. Here's a quick way to measure your risk: Look at your belt. According to the National Institutes of Health, a waist size of over 35 inches in women and over 40 inches in men is linked with much higher disease risk. The good news: For most people, the weight they lose comes off the middle first.

THE BENEFITS OF WEIGHT LOSS

If you're overweight or obese, losing 5–10 percent of your body weight can reliably lower blood pressure, lower triglycerides (blood fats), increase "good" HDL cholesterol (which protects against heart disease), and lower total cholesterol (including "bad" LDL cholesterol), and bring down fasting blood sugar levels even in peo-

What's Your BMI?

Height	BMI 25 (weight in pounds)	BMI 27 (weight in pounds)	BMI 30 (weight in pounds)
4'10"	119	129	143
4'11"	124	133	148
5'	128	138	153
5'1"	132	143	158
5'2"	136	147	164
5'3"	141	152	169
5'4"	145	157	174
5'5"	150	162	180
5'6"	155	167	186
5'7"	159	172	191
5'8"	164	177	197
5'9"	169	182	203
5'10"	174	188	207
5'11"	179	193	215
6'	184	199	221
6'1"	189	204	227
6'2"	194	210	233
6'3	200	216	240
6'4"	205	221	246

ple without diabetes. Such modest weight loss can also reduce abdominal obesity, further lowering your risk of diabetes and heart disease. "You don't have to lose a lot of weight to have a health benefit," says Baylor College of Medicine's John Foreyt. "Five percent to 10 percent is achievable, maintainable, sustainable, whereas 20 percent may not be."

HOW FAST SHOULD YOU LOSE WEIGHT?

Slow and steady really does win this race. Sure, you can drop weight quickly, but it will creep back. Rapid weight loss (more than 2 pounds a week) may increase your risk of gallstones and, possibly, electrolyte abnormalities, which can lead to heart abnormalities in some people. But the worst part is that such rapid weight loss has no long-term benefit. Why? In the year after they've lost weight, slower losers regain just a little weight, while quick losers regain a lot more. Lose weight too quickly, and your metabolism will slow and you'll lose extra lean body mass (muscle), both of which make it easier to regain weight. That's why the NIH recommends relatively slow weight loss: "Many studies show that rapid weight reduction almost always is followed by regaining of weight." Losing weight and regaining it repeatedly, a phenomenon known scientifically as "weight cycling" and popularly as "yo-yo dieting," has not been proven to be unhealthy, but it can certainly be psychologically dispiriting.

The NIH's focus is weight loss methods that have the greatest chance of leading to long-term weight management. The best results come from a combination of a reduced-calorie diet, increased exercise, and behavior modification that helps you stick with your new lifestyle. The goal: *Lose 1–2 pounds a week.*

If you lose weight at that rate, it's not only safe, but can be sustained, week after week. At a pound a week, you can drop 10 pounds in 10 weeks. If you need to lose 25 pounds, that can be achieved over 6 months. You won't feel you are on a "diet," especially if you use the principles in this book to maintain your normal portion sizes. You will develop the eating and physical activity lifestyle that makes permanent weight management possible.

"We used to tell people to go out and lose all the weight they could and then try to maintain that weight loss," says University of Colorado medicine professor James O. Hill, a member of the NIH expert panel. "But that model doesn't work very well. You're constantly fighting against regaining. The new approach is stepwise. You lose up to 10 percent of your body weight over 6 months, and then you work at maintaining that weight loss over the next 6 months."

PLANNING TO LOSE

A weight management program falls into two parts: weight loss and weight loss maintenance. To lose weight, the equation is simple:

Take in fewer calories than you burn. Most of this caloric "deficit" will come from the dietary side: *Reduce intake by about 500 calories a day below what's needed to maintain your current weight.* (See "How Many Calories Do You Need," p. 32)

That should lead to weight loss of about a pound a week. This is appropriate for people who are overweight or moderately obese (BMI of 27 to 35) If you are more severely obese (BMI above 35), you may need to create a caloric deficit of 500 to 1,000 calories so you lose up to 2 pounds a week (because you weigh more, you'll need to lose more pounds to achieve a 10 percent weight loss over six months).

Your diet should be a *Volumetrics* one: low in energy density; rich in complex carbohydrates including fiber-rich whole grains, vegetables, fruits, and beans; adequate in lean sources of protein and low-fat dairy; moderately but not excessively low in fat; with only a few caloric beverages or alcoholic drinks. Our menus (p. 149) are based on 1,600 and 2,000 calories, but they can be adjusted down to 1,400 calories if your calorie needs are lower, or up to 2,400 or more if you are a tall active person, or for the maintenance phase of your weight management plan.

You'll also need to become more physically active. A good exercise program not only increases your metabolic odds of keeping the weight off, it also makes it easier to stick to a healthy lifestyle.

MAINTAIN IT

After about 6 months, weight loss often slows. If you reach such a plateau, this is the time to shift your attention to maintenance. Your goal: to maintain the weight you've lost for the next 6 months, and beyond. You may regain a bit, but you'll work hard at keeping that weight gain to a minimum. If you've lost 25 pounds, and regain only 5 of those pounds over the next 2 years, consider yourself a success.

After 6 months of weight loss, and 6 months of maintenance, you may decide that you want to try to lose more weight. Now is the time to go back to your gradual weight loss program.

How Many Calories Do You Need?

To choose the calorie level of your weight loss plan, you first need to determine how many calories you need per day to maintain your current weight. Then you'll choose a calorie level about 500 calories lower. While many factors influence individual caloric needs—age (caloric needs decline about 2 percent a decade), sex (men tend to be bigger and need more calories), metabolic rate, genetics, and degree of muscularity (muscle requires more calories than fat)—the main ones are how much you weigh now, and how active you are.

You already know your weight. How active are you? You are a "sedentary" person if you do little or no walking, stair climbing, gardening, or other physical activity on a daily basis. To become "moderately active," you'll need to expend about 150 calories a day in physical activity, the equivalent of walking about two miles. Now multiply your weight (in pounds) by the appropriate number below:

Sedentary woman:	12
Sedentary man:	14
Moderately active woman:	15
Moderately active man:	17

Let's say you are a 5′4″ moderately active woman who weighs 157 pounds. Multiply 157 by 15 to get 2,355. That's the number of calories you'll need per day to stay the same weight. To lose a pound a week, you'll need to cut 500 calories a day, bringing your daily caloric intake down to 1,855. To do so, you can follow our 2,000-calorie plan and forgo one 150-calorie snack a day. At that calorie level, you'll lose about a pound a week.

Now it's 12 weeks later and you've lost 12 pounds. You weigh 145. Your BMI has dropped from an overweight 27 to a normal-weight 25. Now work on maintaining that weight loss, to give your body a chance to adjust to this new weight. But don't go back to eating nearly 2,400 calories! Your caloric needs are down, too: 145 times 15 equals about 2,175 calories. That's your new maintenance calorie level.

If you are bigger, or more overweight, your caloric needs will be higher. For example, a man who is 5′11″ and weighs 220 pounds (BMI: 29.5) and is inactive needs 3,080 calories a day (220 pounds times 14). So your weight loss calorie level is about 2,580 (3,080 minus 500 calories). You'll modify our 2,000-calorie plan to reach 2,580 calories. If you lose 25 pounds over the next 6 months, you'll weigh 195 pounds (BMI: 27) and need 2,730 calories (195 times 14). If you have also increased your activity level, you'll be able to eat 3,375 calories a day and stay at your new lower body weight. Your goal now is to maintain that weight for 6 months before contemplating another weight loss effort.

What if you've lost weight over 6 months, and 2 or 3 months later, you find your weight creeping up again? Remember that these are only general guidelines. You'll need to find the pattern that works best for you. Some people find if weight creeps up, it helps to lose it in a few weeks by going back to a weight loss eating style. Let's say you lose 15 pounds but regain 5 over the next 2 months. You can cut back on calories and increase physical activity so you lose that 5 pounds over the next month. *Now* return to the maintenance phase, and strive to keep off the weight over the next 6 months.

To monitor your weight maintenance, you'll need to weigh yourself. We don't recommend daily weighing when you are actively losing weight, because normal daily weight fluctuations can be misleading; a weekly weigh-in, at the same time of the day, without clothes, is a good approach. During the maintenance phase, however, many people who have been successful at losing weight and keeping it off do weigh themselves every day. That way, if you notice that your weight is consistently creeping up over several days or a week, you can make minor changes in your eating and activity habits to prevent further weight gain, or take off a pound or two. That's easier than discovering that you've gained 5 or 10 pounds, and trying to lose it again.

The main shift in thinking is away from quick weight loss to *sustainable* weight loss. You should feel as good about yourself for keeping lost weight off as for losing it in the first place. Maintenance is where most dieters fail. But you don't have to. You will have found a *Volumetrics* eating style that's enjoyable, and will experience the emotional as well as physical benefits of exercise. As the National Institutes of Health's guidelines put it, "The longer the weight maintenance phase can be sustained, the better the prospects for long-term success in weight reduction."

A HEALTHY APPROACH

Losing weight by eating the *Volumetrics* way and increasing your daily physical activity will improve your health. You'll actually start getting healthier from the very first day, before you lose an ounce. This way of eating is nutritionally well balanced, with more than adequate amounts of protein, minerals, and vitamins, and it's a dietary pattern that's been shown to reduce heart disease and other risks.

Exercise will also make you healthier. Even if you didn't lose a pound (don't worry, you will), increasing your level of physical activity can lower your risk of having a heart attack or stroke, raise "good" HDL cholesterol and lower "bad" LDL cholesterol, improve circulation, reduce blood pressure, improve blood sugar control, and reduce the risk of developing type 2 diabetes. If you include weight-bearing exercise like walking, you'll reduce your risk of developing osteoporosis. "Much of the health risk we see in overweight and obese men can be accounted for by their low fitness," says Steven Blair, director of research at the Cooper Institute in Dallas. "Whether you are thin or obese, being active and fit provides important benefits in terms of longevity." Getting more active is also the best way to maintain weight loss. Says Baylor's John Foreyt, "You can lose weight without exercising, but you can't keep it off." (For our exercise program, see "The Exercise Prescription," p. 258.)

SUMMARY

- Be optimistic. You can lose weight and keep it off.

- Choose a realistic weight loss goal. If you are overweight, losing 5 percent to 10 percent of your body weight is achievable and sustainable.

- Being overweight or obese increases your risk of heart disease, diabetes, and other chronic conditions. If you carry your weight around your waist, or already have risk factors such as high blood pressure, the health risks associated with obesity are even greater.

- Losing 5 percent to 10 percent of your body weight can substantially lower these health risks.

- The best way to lose weight is to consume 500 fewer calories a day while increasing physical activity. That will lead to a weight loss of about a pound a week.

- If you have a lot of weight to lose, you may need a 1,000-calorie deficit to lose about 2 pounds a week.

- Losing 1–2 pounds a week is the best rate for long-term success. Lose weight faster, and you'll simply regain much of it.

- Plan to lose weight at this rate for up to 6 months, depending on how much you need to lose. Then focus on weight loss maintenance: sensible *Volumetric* eating and increased physical exercise.

A balanced, varied low-energy-dense dietary pattern, combined with increased physical activity, will improve your health.

Seven Keys to Weight Management Success

The combined intervention of a low calorie diet, increased physical activity, and behavior therapy provides the most successful therapy for weight loss and weight maintenance.
— NATIONAL INSTITUTES OF HEALTH
CLINICAL GUIDELINES FOR THE
TREATMENT OF OVERWEIGHT AND OBESITY

Long-term weight management requires new eating and activity habits. Yet change takes effort. After all, if you're forty and eat five meals and snacks a day, you've done so 70,000 times by now. Fortunately, weight management experts have developed behavior modification approaches that are proven to make permanent lifestyle change easier. If you employ these techniques, the chances are you'll lose more weight than if you simply try to change your eating and exercise habits. You'll also increase your chances of keeping the weight off. Here are the seven most effective "behavior mod" strategies:

1 **Keep a food and exercise log.** "It's absolutely critical," says Baylor's John Foreyt. Keeping food records is the best predictor of successful weight loss in several studies. People who keep exercise logs are also more likely to stick with their exercise programs.

   Write down what you eat at each meal or snack during the day, with approximate serving sizes. Now look for ways to substitute foods of lower energy density, and make gradual changes. For example, if your breakfast is an energy-dense Danish pastry, try an English muffin with jam. Now write down how you feel after making these changes. That way, you'll identify which foods taste best and best curb hunger. In the same book, keep a daily log of when you engage in physical activity, what you do, how long, and how intensely. Record how you felt before you took a brisk walk, for example, and afterward. Write down any obstacles to becoming more active, and your ideas for overcoming them.

2 **Identify and manage cues for overeating and underactivity.** If you find certain foods (such as chocolate, cookies, cheese, or chips) hard not to overeat, keep them out of the house entirely, and eat them only on special occasions in a restaurant or food shop. Or decide to eat only in certain rooms of the house, such as the dining room, rather than in the living room in front of the television. Create an environment where it's easier to stick to moderation.

   "Put yourself in situations where you can have a favorite food but not overeat," says Foreyt. "Don't buy a pound of chocolate, buy two pieces, and take them home with you. That's a situation where you won't binge." Structure your environment so you eat only at certain times. "If I had a bowl of chocolate chip cookies in front on me, I'd be nibbling on them now," admits Foreyt. "But I've learned to keep food away from me when it's not time to eat."

3 **Work on your thoughts and feelings.** Psychologists call this "cognitive restructuring": learning to interpret events and expectations in a more constructive way. Unrealistic weight loss goals, or expectations that weight loss will solve all your problems, can lead to self-defeating thoughts and feelings that can undermine weight loss efforts. Realistic goals and expectations can set you up for success. You'll also

want to work on how to interpret less-than-ideal food choices. For example, if you have a donut on the way to work, you might think, "Oh, now I've really blown it; I might as well eat whatever I want today." A more constructive thought: "Okay, so I ate a donut, but if I make healthier choices at lunch and dinner, I'll still wind up with a good eating day."

4 **Learn stress management.** Many people overeat in response to stress. But if you are eating in response to stress, it's easy to override satiety signals. That's why it's so important to learn how to calm down first, before you react by overeating. Deep breathing, progressive muscle relaxation, and meditation are all effective. So is exercise.

5 **Get involved with family and friends.** People who have more social support do better in weight management. Examples: Ask a family member to go on a *Volumetrics* menu plan with you, enter a weight control program with a friend, or join a weight loss support group or a program such as Weight Watchers that encourages a support system. You could also begin walking regularly with a friend, or join a mall walking club. Social support needn't be weight-related to be helpful. "Work on relationships," says Foreyt. "Volunteer. I tell my students to take classes—sailing, bridge, anything. Any time you get involved with other people, you start prioritizing things. You find that people are more important than food. As you build relationships, you'll be less likely to use food as a comfort."

6 **Move!** "When obese people start exercising, they feel better about themselves, and that feeling really helps them stick to a healthy lifestyle," says Foreyt. "Even if you didn't burn a single calorie, you'd have to exercise for the feeling of well-being. We all work so hard, we need to feel good."

7 **Make a plan to handle setbacks.** No one loses weight every day for months; some weeks are better than others. It's not just about eating a high-calorie food one day; you *should* include small portions of energy-dense favorite foods in your eating plan. Even if you overindulge, realize that it's normal, and move on.

Plan ahead for social situations that may trigger "relapses": holiday parties, family vacations, even emotional upsets. Think ahead about how you will handle each of these situations. And if you do find yourself overeating, ask yourself, "What did I learn from this experience? What can I do differently the next time?" Give yourself positive reinforcement, such as nonfood rewards for sticking to your plan.

Should you do it yourself? By all means, if that's your style. Just under half of people who've successfully lost weight and kept it off do it on their own, while others join a program. Weight Watchers, Jenny Craig, and TOPS (Take Off Pounds Sensibly), for example, have each recently joined the Federal Trade Commission (FTC) Partnership for Healthy Weight Management, and agree to voluntarily disclose essential information to consumers; they are all sensible programs, and consistent with *Volumetrics*.

Another excellent option is to work with a nutritionist who has an M.S. or Ph.D. or is a registered dietician (R.D.); these people are trained to help you not only choose a healthier diet, but apply these behavioral techniques that help make lifestyle changes stick. To find an R.D., contact the American Dietetic Association (see "Resources," p. 300). Bring a copy of this book to the first meeting, and your nutrition counselor can help you put *Volumetrics* into practice.

FOOD AND BEVERAGE CHOICES play a major role in determining how easy it will be to control calories. We'll help you make smart choices by exploring five major components of the diet:

- **Fat.** Whether solid at room temperature (butter) or liquid (canola oil), visible (marbling in steak) or invisible (in sauce), fats are the most energy dense of all food components. If you eat a moderately low-fat diet (20–30 percent of calories), you'll be able to eat satisfying portions while managing your weight.

- **Carbohydrates.** Bread, rice, pasta, corn, potatoes, dry beans, other vegetables, fruits, and table sugar all derive most or all their calories from carbohydrate, which includes both sugar (simple molecules) and starch (longer chain molecules). Fiber is made of long chains of molecules that we can't digest. You can enhance satiety on fewer calories by selecting carbohydrate-rich foods high in water content and fiber and low in energy density.

- **Protein.** Beef, pork, lamb, chicken, turkey, fish, shellfish, dry beans and peas, soy products, and dairy products are all rich in protein, which is composed of amino acids our bodies need to build muscle and make biological compounds. Protein is particularly satiating, so make sure you eat normal portions of lean protein foods whether you are losing weight or preventing weight gain.

- **Alcohol.** Beer, wine, and spirits contain alcohol (ethanol), a byproduct of fermentation. Alcohol is almost as energy dense as fat, and is also, of course, intoxicating. Alcoholic beverages add calories while providing little satiety, but there are ways to include them while controlling calories.

- **Water** is a simple molecule with no calories. The amount of water in a food is a crucial influence on its energy density. Consuming water-rich foods is a core strategy for lowering your diet's energy density. But simply drinking more water won't help with satiety.

Lowering the energy density of the foods you eat is critical for controlling hunger as you manage your weight. As we tour the major components of the diet we'll show you what this means for specific food choices. In the last chapter in this section, we'll look at a case study—soup—to show you how a low-energy-dense food helps you feel full on fewer calories.

Fat

Many's the long night I've dreamed of cheese—
toasted, mostly.
—ROBERT LOUIS STEVENSON,
Treasure Island, 1883

IF YOU EAT A CLASSIC HIGH-FAT American diet, learning to lower the fat content of your overall diet is an essential step in your weight management program. With 9 calories per gram, fat can pack a lot of calories into even small portions. This, combined with the delicious effects fat can have on foods, makes it very easy to overeat high-fat foods. Cutting the fat in your diet is crucial if you want to lower the energy density of your diet and eat the *Volumetrics* way.

Yet fat's role in weight management has been overblown. The main reason Americans are gaining weight is that we consume more calories than we burn up in physical activity and metabolism. *Any* excess calories will lead to weight gain, whether they come from carbohydrates, protein, fat, or alcohol.

The reason you need to decrease the amount of fat you eat for weight management is that this will reduce the overall energy density of your diet, so you can eat normal-size portions. If you try to cut calories without cutting fat, you'll need to eat portions so small that you'll be hungry. That's why we recommend a moderately low-fat diet that gets 20–30 percent of its calories from fat: You can eat enough food to stay satisfied.

Fat makes food taste better. While some fat-free foods are naturally delicious—a juicy ripe peach, a garden tomato, a blackberry sorbet—others, like cookies, cake, and cheese, can sometimes resemble cardboard or rubber when their moistening, flavor-carrying fat is removed. Ironically, both a high-fat diet and a very low-fat diet can undermine efforts to stick to a calorie-controlled eating plan: Too much fat means too little food, but too little fat can mean taste deprivation, and deprivation backfires. Cut fat intelligently, and you'll be able to eat plenty of food, enjoy it as much as ever, and still control calories.

WHY WE OVEREAT HIGH-FAT FOODS

High-fat diets promote obesity. We know that. But why? Are the reasons related to taste, metabolism, or calories? Each plays a role, as we'll show you, but a major reason that high-fat foods are easy to overeat is that they pack a lot of calories in a small portion.

What Is Fat?

Fats, large molecules in food, serve as building blocks for important compounds in the body, but their primary role is as a concentrated source of calories. The various types of fat are equally caloric.

They do have different health effects; however, particularly on the cardiovascular system. Saturated fats, found mostly in fatty red meat and high-fat dairy foods, increase heart disease risk by raising blood cholesterol. So do trans fats, found in foods that list "partially hydrogenated oils" as an ingredient: hard margarine (soft or liquid ones are okay), many commercial baked goods, and fried foods. By contrast, plant and fish oils—found in fish and seafood, olive and canola oils, and nuts and seeds—are made up of unsaturated fats that reduce heart disease risk. If you eat fewer foods high in saturated and trans fats, while including small amounts of foods rich in unsaturated fats, you can eat less total fat, lower energy density, and improve health.

How Much Fat Can I Eat?

Typically Americans eat 30–40 percent of their calories from fat. The best range for both weight control and health is 20–30 percent. Why? A low-fat diet helps prevent weight gain, and helps lower the energy density of foods. If you're consuming a high-fat diet, cutting back to 30 percent will mean you can eat bigger portions. Indeed, the less fat in your diet, the more you can eat for the same calories. So you may want to aim lower, to 25 percent of calories from fat. At 20 percent, you'll be able to eat even more. If you go further, to 15 percent or 10 percent or lower, however, you'll probably find that you have to cut out so many tasty foods that your new dietary pattern will be hard to sustain as a lifestyle. Because our goal is to help you find a way of eating that will help you feel satisfied with a lower-calorie eating style permanently, we don't advise such an extreme approach.

AMOUNT OF FAT (IN GRAMS) YOU CAN EAT AT EACH DAILY CALORIE LEVEL

Daily Calories	30 Percent of Calories from Fat	25 Percent Fat	20 Percent Fat
1,200	40	33	27
1,600	53	44	36
2,000	67	56	44
2,400	80	67	53

Let's look at some examples of how fat increases energy density and affects the amount of food you can eat. Suppose you want bread with dinner. For 140 calories, you can have 2 large slices of French bread—it has only 1 gram of fat. But if you want 2 teaspoons of butter containing 8 grams of fat, you can have only 1 slice (*figure A*, next page). (We abbreviate "energy density" as E.D. in these illustrations.)

Or consider how fat affects a serving of baked potato. By itself, a baked potato is a food of low energy density. A medium baked potato (2½ inches by 4¾ inches) weighing 6½ ounces has only about 200 calories and no fat. To stay at that calorie level when you top it with 2 tablespoons of regular high-fat sour cream containing 5 grams of fat, you can eat only ¾ of the potato. With a tablespoon

Figure A: 140 Calories of Bread

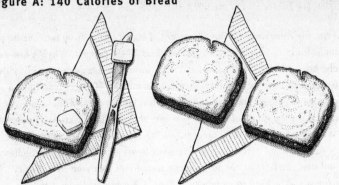

French bread with 2 teaspoons of butter. E.D.: 4.0. Serving size: 1 slice.

French bread without a spread. E.D.: 2.75. Serving size: 2 slices.

High-fat foods like butter are very energy dense: Two teaspoons have the same number of calories as a slice of bread.

Figure B: 200 Calories of Potato

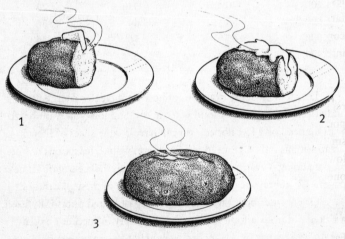

1

2

3

1 *Baked potato with 1 tablespoon butter. E.D.: 1.9. Serving size: ½ potato.*

2 *Baked potato with 2 tablespoons regular sour cream. E.D.: 1.2. Serving size: ¾ potato.*

3 *Baked potato. E.D.: 1.1. Serving size: 1 potato.*

A little butter or sour cream has the same calories as a lot of potato!

of butter, you only get half a potato and 12 grams of fat. Note how the serving size decreases as the fat content increases *(figure B)*.

Does this mean you should only eat a baked potato with nothing on it? Of course not. It's up to you to make the choice. You could choose 1 tablespoon of full-fat sour cream, or stick with 2 tablespoons but choose low-fat sour cream, perhaps mixed with salsa. Or you might decide that you really want "real" sour cream or butter on your potato. Just make sure that you eat a smaller portion.

As a scientist, I (Barbara) didn't always believe that fat's main contribution to overeating was its ability to pack a lot of calories in a small portion. I, along with other researchers in the field, believed that fat was inherently less satiating than protein or carbohydrate. We researchers thought fat could sneak in unnoticed by the regulatory systems in our bodies that are designed to stop eating. Many reviews of satiety indicate that there is a hierarchy of satiety, with protein being the most satiating, then carbohydrate, and finally, pulling up the caboose, fat. There is evidence that protein *is* more satiating than the other nutrients. But a number of controlled studies in our lab and in England, France, and the Netherlands find that fat and carbohydrate have similar effects on satiety when they are consumed in foods with similar energy densities. Fat does not sneak into our bodies unnoticed by systems regulating satiety.

In the real world, to be sure, fat is often found in foods with a high energy density. Even a small amount of fat—a pat of butter, regular salad dressing—can dramatically increase the calories in a portion of food. If you want to eat those foods, you'll need to eat smaller portions. That reinforces the basic advice of this book to lower the energy density of your dietary pattern. Moderating fat is one part of the *Volumetrics* strategy.

WHY DO WE LOVE FAT SO MUCH?

Fat does many wonderful things to food. It enhances texture, flavor, appearance, and overall palatability. It carries, releases, and enhances flavors coming from the other ingredients in a food, and is a key element in making foods flaky, crispy, crunchy, smooth, hard or soft, oily or juicy.

We learn to like high-fat foods at a young age. In children, a preference for high-fat foods develops quickly. Children learn to like high-fat foods in large part because they are energy dense, and rapidly reduce hunger. "Children learn to prefer foods that are good sources of calories, whether they're from fat or carbohydrates," says Penn State professor Leann Birch. She's found that children quickly learn to favor energy-dense snacks over snacks of lower energy density—whether those extra calories come from fat or carbohydrates. We just learn that energy-dense foods curb hunger quickly. Many of these foods are high in fat, and taste very good.

Fast forward to adulthood. If you're like most Americans, you've grown up liking high-fat, energy-dense foods. This preference for fat is particularly notable in overweight people. "Obesity is associated more with a 'fat tooth' than a 'sweet tooth,'" says University of Washington professor Adam Drewnowski. "Obese women like fat more than sugar, while leaner women like sugar more than fat." Obese men like high-fat foods, too, finds Drewnowski, although the kinds of high-fat foods they prefer are different. "Women like desserts such as chocolate and ice cream more, while men like fat/protein/salt combinations—main dishes like hamburgers, pizza, and hot dogs, and salty snacks."

In short, a liking for high-fat foods, which has its roots in childhood, is a problem for many adults who are trying to control weight. Don't worry, later in this chapter we will tell you how to lower your fat intake while still eating foods you enjoy.

AREN'T FAT CALORIES MORE FATTENING?

There's another reason that weight control experts often advise people to reduce the fat in their diets: A high-fat diet is particularly easy to convert into body fat. Keep in mind, though, that this is a modest effect, and it only affects weight *gain*, not weight loss. If you cut calories below what's needed to maintain your body weight, you'll lose weight no matter what the fat content of your diet is.

On the other hand, if you consume more calories than you need, you'll gain weight no matter what you eat, but you'll gain

Where the Fats Are

To cut fat and lower energy density, it helps to know where the fats are. Here are the major sources of fat in the American diet. We've also provided some suggestions for alternatives.

SOURCES OF FAT	TIPS
Beef and other meats	Buy select, not choice cuts; trim well; cook with little added fat; buy low-fat processed meats.
Margarine and butter	Use less butter; if you use margarine, buy reduced-calorie soft tub or liquid.
Salad dressing/ mayonnaise	Use low-fat or fat-free dressings; try naturally fat-free vinegar or lemon juice.
Cheese	Buy lower-fat cheeses like part-skim mozzarella.
Milk	Use skim or 1 percent.
Cakes/cookies/quick breads/donuts	Look for low-fat or fat-free versions, but watch calories: Many are as energy-dense as the high-fat products they replace; eat less.
Poultry	Remove the skin after baking or broiling. Eat fried chicken infrequently.
Oils	Switch to healthier oils, such as olive or canola; use in moderation; try a spray for cooking and baking.
Potato chips/corn chips/popcorn	Try baked chips, low-fat potato chips, air-popped popcorn with little added fat; watch calories, as these are often as energy-dense as the products they replace.
Eggs	The fat is in the yolk; replace some yolks with egg whites; use egg substitutes.
Nuts/seeds	These provide beneficial fats, so enjoy small amounts.
Ice cream/frozen yogurt	Choose low-fat or fat-free versions, but watch calories, too.

more weight on a high-fat rather than a high-carbohydrate diet. The main reason is that the body is less efficient at converting excess carbohydrate calories into body fat than it is at converting excess calories from fat. If you take in 250 extra calories every day as carbohydrates, you'll gain about 17 pounds of body fat each year. If those calories come from fat, you'll gain about 19 pounds.

We know this is confusing research for many people. It confuses scientists, who often don't make the distinction between weight loss and weight gain. "A low-fat diet is key for the prevention of weight gain," says University of Colorado medicine professor James O. Hill, "but for weight loss, it doesn't matter what you eat, as long as the calories are low." Consider:

- If calories are low enough, you can lose weight even on a high-fat diet. We don't recommend this, but it proves the point. In Swiss research, a 1,000-calorie-a-day weight loss diet was as successful whether fat contributed 25 percent or 53 percent of calories.

- Cutting fat helps to lower calorie intake. When women cut their fat calories from 39 to 22 percent in the Women's Health Trial in the United States, total calories also fell and the women lost weight. By cutting fat they reduced the energy density of their diet and were satisfied on fewer calories.

- A low-fat diet helps prevent weight regain. In Denmark, women who maintained a low-fat lifestyle regained little of the weigh they had lost.

- American women who have successfully lost more than 30 pounds and kept it off for at least a year averaged 24 percent of calories from fat, according to the National Weight Control Registry at the University of Pittsburgh. In *Volumetrics* we recommend that you eat 20–30 percent of your calories from fat.

Calories count. The best way to take in fewer calories is to lower your diet's energy density. But if you do so while consuming a diet that is moderately low in fat—you don't have to go to extremes—you'll improve your chances of keeping the weight off.

If, while losing weight, you eat your normal high-fat foods, but simply restrict your eating, you won't learn habits that will sustain you. When you go back to eating your previous portions of high-fat, energy-dense foods, you'll regain weight.

So make smart lower-fat food choices, as part of an overall *Volumetrics* strategy of lowering the energy density of your diet. You can maintain enough fat in your foods to enjoy the taste and texture it gives them.

CAN YOU LEARN TO LIKE LOW-FAT FOODS?

Like many of you, I (Barbara) have made changes in my diet aimed at reducing fat intake. Over several years I worked my way down from full-fat milk to 2 percent to 1 percent, and now finally I am drinking fat-free skim milk. And I like it! Full-fat milk tastes like cream to me, and I reject the half and half that is forced on me in virtually every restaurant in America. Does this mean that I have become truly fat phobic—that I avoid fat in every food I encounter?

It doesn't work that way. I still like full-fat premium ice cream, another dairy product. And I love chocolate. Fat contributes to the pleasure we get from foods in so many different ways, it may not be possible to get to the point where you can say honestly that you don't like any high-fat foods. Oh, there may be exceptions. If the grim reaper is knocking at your door, and you convince yourself that it is fat that's killing you, maybe you'll change your preferences. But it's not even clear that this occurs. In the program sponsored by Dean Ornish, participants with coronary heart disease are restricted to a 10 percent fat diet. They have to comply or they are ousted from the program. Yet they still dream about their favorite, now forbidden, fatty foods, according to people who run these programs. Even Ornish himself loves chocolate gelato and truffles, and allows himself a very small taste almost every day.

Systematic studies of the fat preferences of women in a long-term fat reduction program reinforce the difficulty of changing the preference for fat. After participants in the Women's Health Trial had been on a 20 percent fat diet for 3 years, they reported that they developed a dislike for the taste of fat, and even felt physically uncomfortable after eating high-fat foods. Yet when researchers at the Fred Hutchinson Cancer Research Center in Seattle offered them high-fat snacks, they ate as many as did women who weren't restricting fat!

So work with it. Focus on dietary changes that reduce fat and energy density in the easiest, most pleasant ways.

SIX WAYS TO EAT LESS FAT

Each of you has your own personal selection of foods you dislike, foods you like, and foods that you like so much they prompt you to overeat. So no one strategy for fat reduction will work for everyone. But researchers such as Alan Kristal at the Hutchinson Center have found that certain changes are particularly easy for most people to make in their diets, and even more important, to keep doing for years. There are six main strategies. The first two are the easiest:

- **Substitute lower-fat versions for high-fat versions of frequently eaten foods.** This includes using low-calorie mayonnaise, low-fat salad dressing, low-fat soups, low-fat cheeses, skim milk, reduced-fat or fat-free sour cream, and low-fat ice cream or frozen yogurt.

- **Reduce the fat in your meat.** This includes trimming the fat from steaks, removing the skin on poultry, buying leaner cuts of beef and pork, and broiling or baking instead of frying. Lean hamburger is available, as is lean ground turkey. Lean luncheon meats are easy to find and taste good.

To reduce fat further, you'll need to try these approaches:

- **Reduce the use of fat as a flavoring.** This one is harder for many people. Do you automatically put sour cream on your potatoes, butter or margarine on your green beans or toast, and gravy on your turkey? Learning different flavoring techniques can greatly lower your fat intake. Experiment with other flavorings: lemon zest on rice, lime juice on fish, orange juice on pork, tomato salsa on baked chicken, balsamic vinegar on salads, malt vinegar on beans, low-fat or nonfat yogurt or sour cream on baked potatoes, prepared mustards on beef and chicken. It's not a question of all or nothing: You can learn to enjoy fish poached in white wine and water with some spices, and still use a small amount of butter or margarine on your bread.

- **Minimize fried foods.** This relates primarily to eating out. At home, instead of frying, try stir-frying in a nonstick pan with a vegetable cooking spray, "dry" sautéing (a skinless chicken breast goes into a preheated nonstick pan with no added fat), sautéing in a little water, cooking in a microwave, stewing, braising, broiling, grilling or roasting (put meats on a rack so fat drips down).

- **Replace high-fat foods with fruits and vegetables.** Having a carrot instead of chips, or an apple instead of apple pie, is a great idea nutritionally, and a great way to cut calories and fat, but it's hard for many people to do. One way to make it easier is to search out fruits and vegetables you really like.

- **Eat more grains, vegetables, beans, and fruit, and less meat, dairy, and baked goods.** This basic change from a meat- and dairy-centered diet to one that is more plant-based is one that nutritionists strongly recommend to reduce the risk of chronic disease, yet it's also one of the hardest changes to make. But the more you can make the transition toward a plant-based diet, with smaller portions of lean red meats and poultry and fish, and larger portions of grains, beans, fruits, and vegetables, the more you'll be able to cut fat from your diet. You'll also be greatly lowering the energy density of your diet, which in the end is more important for weight management.

The Milk Strategy

What's one of the easiest ways to cut fat in your diet? It may be to simply choose a lower-fat milk. In a Food and Drug Administration study of 15,000 Americans, those who chose low-fat (1%) or fat-free milk consumed the least total fat in their diet. Research at Penn State reveals that nearly every successful dietary strategy for lowering fat intake included drinking lower-fat milk. Because milk fat is mostly saturated, cutting that fat not only lowers calories in your diet, but also helps lower cholesterol. You'll also lower the energy density of your glass of milk, which means you'll be able to either drink more, or drink the same amount and consume fewer calories. For 100 calories, you can either drink just over a half cup of whole milk or more than a cup of skim milk. A cup, by the way, has 8 ounces.

100 Calories of Milk

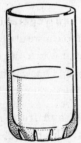

Whole Milk. E.D.: 0.6. Serving Size: 5⅓ ounces.

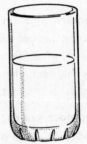

Reduced-Fat (2%) Milk. E.D.: 0.5. Serving Size: 6⅔

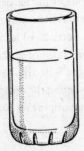

Low-Fat (1%) Milk. E.D.: 0.4. Serving Size: 7¾ ounces.

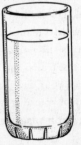

Fat-Free (Skim) Milk. E.D.: 0.35. Serving Size: 9¼ ounces.

WHAT ABOUT FAT SUBSTITUTES?

For most people their biggest fear in trying to lose weight is the prospect of giving up their favorite foods. And let's face it, changing your eating habits is very difficult. This is why the easiest fat-reduction strategy is to substitute reduced-fat or nonfat foods for the full-fat version. This strategy works best if you can find a reduced-fat food that tastes as good, or almost as good, as the full-fat food it replaces. This is where fat substitutes can play an important role in *Volumetrics*. They can reduce the energy density of a wide range of foods.

Many people misunderstand what fat substitutes are and lump them together as synthetic and unhealthy. But a fat substitute is any ingredient that is used to replace the fat in foods. This can be done with natural ingredients such as applesauce. There are also many different types of commercial fat substitutes in a wide range of products. They may be made from common food ingredients, used in slightly different ways. Proteins and various carbohydrates, including soluble fibers, can mimic the sensory characteristics of fat. Fat substitutes made from carbohydrates or proteins contain some calories, though less than the fat they are replacing. Often only small amounts are needed to improve the sensory quality of products. Here's an example of how you can use a typical reduced-fat product such as salad dressing, made with carbohydrate-based fat substitutes, to lower a salad's energy density, allowing you to eat fewer calories in your usual size portion.

You've prepared a *Volumetric* salad, with a cup and a half of leaf lettuce. The lettuce has only 15 calories, yet fills up a bowl. But watch how your choice of salad dressing affects the total calories in your salad. Let's suppose that you add 2 tablespoons of dressing containing 170 calories. If you substitute fat-free dressing for the full-fat version, you will save 120 calories and 18 grams of fat. Or you may prefer to use a reduced-fat dressing. This will save you 60 calories and 7 grams of fat in the 2 tablespoons. Of course, another option is to try cutting back on the amount of full-fat dressing you are using. You may find you like the salad with less dressing.

Recently, a synthetic fat substitute with zero fat and calories was approved for use in a limited range of snack foods. The fat substitute olestra (marketed as Olean) gives foods the taste and texture of fat, but cannot be absorbed, so it passes out of the body undigested. Because it adds bulk to foods, it lowers not only fat but also the energy density. For example, if you substitute fat-free potato chips made with olestra for full-fat chips, you will cut calories in half. But you still need to watch portions. Even fat-free chips are fairly energy dense.

There have been health concerns that olestra causes vitamin losses and gastrointestinal upset. As olestra passes out of the body it carries with it fat-soluble vitamins (A, D, E, and K, and carotenoids) from foods eaten at about the same time. The fat-soluble vitamins are added back to olestra-containing foods, but carotenoids and other phytochemicals, the health-promoting compounds found in many fruits and vegetables, aren't replaced. To minimize the loss of these compounds, you may want to eat your fruits and vegetables at least an hour before or after you consume olestra-containing snacks. The abdominal cramping and diarrhea that have been widely reported were not seen in several well-controlled trials in which the participants did not know they were eating olestra-containing foods.

If you have concerns about any fat substitutes, you do not need to include them in your diet. Because fat substitutes offer potential to lower the energy density of foods while preserving their taste, you may decide to include some in your diet. If so, and you have not tried a particular substitute before, we recommend that you try a small portion and see what happens. It is never a good idea to eat a large amount of a food you have never tried.

Do fat substitutes really help with weight management? They do help cut fat intake. Studies in the United States, England, France, and the Netherlands consistently found that when people consumed foods made with olestra, they ate less fat over the day—they didn't get a "craving" for fatty foods later. But it's not clear whether fat substitutes help people lower their total calories and lose weight. In some studies, olestra helped people eat fewer calories; in others, participants made up the calories at later meals. Large-scale trials of the effects of olestra on body weight are in progress.

So the jury is still out. But it is clear that substituting a bag of low-fat or fat-free chips for full-fat chips once a week won't help much with weight management. On the other hand, as part of a multipronged total dietary plan, foods made with fat substitutes can play a role. You'll have a wider range of reduced-calorie foods from which to choose. Substituting fat-free or lower-fat versions for high-fat versions of frequently eaten foods only works if you don't give yourself a license to eat more snacks and sweets. Before buying a fat-modified snack or sweet, ask yourself, "Would I be eating this if it weren't fat-free or low-fat?" If not, you may simply be adding those calories to your dietary total. On the other hand, if you'd be eating chips or cookies anyway, and switch to a fat-free or lower-fat version, and *eat the same amount*, you may be saving yourself both fat and calories. *Read food labels carefully to make sure that lower-fat foods are also lower in calories.*

Choosing foods that are reduced in fat is a key strategy in *Volumetrics*. It allows you to reduce the energy density of your diet so you can enjoy satisfying portions. We emphasize the importance of the amount of fat you eat because fat has such a high energy density, but moderating your fat intake is only one of your strategies to find a way of eating that gives you plenty of good-tasting food without too many calories. In the following chapters, you'll learn more *Volumetrics* strategies.

SUMMARY

- Decreasing the fat content of your diet will lower its energy density and allow you to eat satisfying portions.

- High-fat foods are easy to overeat because they are energy dense and taste good.

- Excess fat calories are easily converted to body fat. This is another reason that high-fat diets lead to weight gain.

- For weight loss it is calorie reduction that matters. If you eat fewer calories than you need, you will lose weight no matter what the fat content. But a low-fat, low-energy-dense diet will satisfy your hunger better.

- While fat is energy dense, the solution isn't to shun fat, but to moderate it, and focus on lowering the overall energy density of your dietary pattern. This will help you to reduce calories.

- You can decrease your preference for fat in some foods, such as milk. The more reduced-fat foods you can learn to like, the greater your chances for permanently lowering your fat intake.

- The two easiest ways for most people to cut fat are to substitute lower-fat versions of frequently eaten foods for high-fat counterparts, and to reduce the fat in the meat they eat. Try other methods too: Find alternatives to fat as a flavoring, minimize fried foods, replace high-fat foods with fruits and vegetables, and eat more grains, vegetables, and fruit.

- Make sure that reduced-fat foods are also lower in calories than the regular versions.

- For fat-free or reduced-fat foods to help cut both fat and calories, you need to use them as true substitutes for the higher-fat counterpart. Don't give yourself a license to eat more.

Carbohydrates

Everything you see, I owe to spaghetti.
—SOPHIA LOREN

HOW WOULD YOU FEEL if we told you that to achieve permanent weight loss you have to give up eating bread, potatoes, rice, and pasta, not to mention any food high in sugar? Or even if we didn't ask you to give them up altogether, just to cut way back? Our guess is that most of you would say that there is no hope of sticking to such a diet. Yet if the most popular weight loss books are any indication, many of you have tried this strategy.

It really is amazing that there is so much confusion about foods that form the foundation of the human diet. In nutrition surveys, many people label "starchy" foods (pasta, bread, potatoes) as "favorable for weight control," while others call them "fattening." One reason for this perplexity is that popular articles and books have given the public misinformation about carbohydrates and obesity. We'll clear that up.

Our basic message is positive: Carbohydrates have been the mainstay of weight control diets for many years. They still should be. Most of our calories should come from complex carbohydrates, which are found only in plant foods such as grains, potatoes, beans, and vegetables. Fruits, rich in water, fiber, vitamins, and minerals, contain sugars—simple carbohydrates—and also deserve a place on your table.

Carbohydrate sources such as grains, vegetables, and fruit should be the core of your diet. Complement this core with lean sources of protein and low-fat dairy foods. That is the best dietary pattern for both health and weight management.

It's possible to overeat carbohydrate-rich foods, of course. As a nation, we're consuming more calories than ever, and most of those extra calories are coming from carbohydrates. Calories count from any source. The key to preventing such overeating is to choose carbohydrate-rich foods low in energy density that satisfy you without providing too many calories. (We'll look at carbohydrate-containing beverages in "Water and Other Beverages," p. 91.) Here's how high-carbohydrate foods stack up in terms of energy density:

- **Very low-energy-dense foods.** Most fresh fruits and vegetables are very low in energy density.

- **Low-energy-dense foods.** Starchy foods like pasta, cooked grains, potatoes, and legumes (these include dry beans, peas, chickpeas, lima beans, soybeans, and lentils) are low in energy density.

- **Medium-energy-dense foods.** These include fat-free or low-fat, high-carbohydrate snacks such as chips, crackers, pretzels, or sugar-rich foods such as jelly beans; French fries; white bread; and dried fruit.

- **High-energy-dense foods.** Foods high in carbohydrates and fat, such as chocolate bars and potato chips, are high in energy density.

So add volume to your meals with a wide variety of fiber-rich fruits and vegetables. When it comes to lowering the energy density of a meal or snack, these are the real stars.

DOES PASTA MAKE YOU FAT?

The furor over carbohydrates began in earnest in 1995 when the *New York Times* ran a front-page article with the headline, "So It May Be True After All: Eating Pasta Makes You Fat."

The news spread all the way to Italy, where it came as a big surprise. Too many calories from any source, even pasta, can lead to weight gain. But we'd like to let you in on a little secret: *In the real world, people who eat a high proportion of carbohydrates in their diets are less prone to obesity.* That's what large population studies find.

One reason is that if you take in more carbohydrates you're likely to take in less fat—and vice versa. When the fat content goes down, the energy density usually decreases as well. In most cases, a high-carbohydrate diet gives you fewer calories.

Carbohydrates play an important role in *Volumetrics*. Complex carbohydrates, especially whole-grain ones, contain fiber, which bulks up food with few calories. Grains also absorb water, further reducing their energy density. While even a fat-free or low-fat dry carbohydrate snack like a cracker has an energy density of about 4 calories per gram, cooked spaghetti's energy density is only 1.5.

A half-cup of cooked spaghetti has only 65 calories. Leave off high-fat cream-based sauces and instead serve with low-fat tomato-based sauces and vegetables, and the spaghetti's energy density goes lower. To make a complete meal, simply add a modest portion (2–3 ounces) of a protein-rich food such as dry beans, lean meats, poul-

What Are Carbohydrates?
Starch, Fiber, and Sugars

Grains, bread, cereals, vegetables, fruits, and table sugar are all primarily carbohydrates, the nutrient that serves as the body's main fuel. There are two main types: complex carbohydrates and simple carbohydrates. Fiber is a form of carbohydrate that cannot be digested. All carbohydrates are made up of units of simple sugars joined together.

Simple carbohydrates are sugars. The term *sugars* refers to all sweet carbohydrates, such as glucose, fructose, and sucrose. *Sugar* refers just to sucrose (table sugar). Some sugars occur naturally in fruits and even vegetables, but many more are added to foods, with ingredient names including brown sugar, corn sweetener, corn syrup, fructose, fruit juice concentrate, glucose (dextrose), high-fructose corn syrup, honey, invert sugar, lactose, maltose, molasses, raw sugar, table sugar (sucrose), and syrup. If any one of these is the first or second ingredient in a food, or if several of them are listed, that food is high in added sugars.

Complex carbohydrates are composed primarily of *starch*—large molecules made up of long chains of sugars. Between half and three-quarters of the weight of a grain like wheat or rice is starch; half a potato by weight is starch.

Fiber is not a source of calories. It passes undigested into the intestines, adding bulk to stools. Some fibers are insoluble in water, while others are soluble. Insoluble fibers, found in whole wheat and wheat bran as well as vegetable skins, improve bowel function. Soluble fibers, found in fruits, vegetables, oats, and dry beans, lower blood cholesterol. Because of these different health benefits, it's a good idea to eat a wide variety of whole grains, vegetables, and fruits to get both types of fiber.

---

try, fish, seafood, or low-fat cheese. The same principle applies to rice, wheat bread, couscous, cornmeal, oats, barley, rye, or any other grain; starchy vegetables like potatoes, sweet potatoes and corn can also serve as the low-energy-dense core of a meal.

In southern Italy, where pasta is a mainstay, the traditional diet is associated with health and leanness. Pasta is served as a small first course, usually followed by a protein-rich course like fish, with plenty of vegetables, and dessert is often simply a piece of perfectly ripe fruit. That southern Italian dietary pattern gets about 25 percent of its calories from fat, 15 percent from protein, and 60 percent from carbohydrates. Despite this high carbohydrate intake, obesity is rarer in Italy than in the United States.

Weight loss diets that limit high-carbohydrate staple foods such as bread and potatoes greatly restrict your food choices, and that is why you'll eat fewer calories. When you eat very little carbohydrate and lots of protein, your body also responds by shedding water, so you will lose weight. But you haven't lost body fat, which is what matters. When you eat normally again, the water weight returns quickly. A low-carbohydrate diet is not optimal for health and is hard to sustain.

THE INSULIN CONNECTION

Many popular books now argue that carbohydrates contribute to obesity not just through their calories, but also by stimulating insulin secretion, which promotes body fat. It's true that carbohydrates stimulate insulin secretion. This controls the process by which carbohydrates, which are composed of chains of sugars, are broken down into blood sugar (glucose). In people with normal insulin responses, only a small amount of insulin is needed to regulate this process. "Insulin does not make you gain weight," says Stanford University professor of medicine Gerald Reaven. Carefully controlled metabolic studies confirm that we should worry a lot less about a carbohydrate/insulin/obesity connection. People do not gain weight on a high-carbohydrate diet *unless they are eating excess calories*.

But what about people who don't have a normal response to insulin? Their cells are not sensitive to the insulin signal, so the pancreas has to secrete extra insulin to control blood sugar. They are "insulin resistant." Insulin resistance is often seen in overweight people, especially those who are also sedentary.

But it wasn't insulin resistance that made them obese and it wasn't eating lots of carbohydrates that led to insulin resistance in the first place. Instead, excess calories, excess weight, and lack of physical activity led to the insulin resistance. In rural China, Japan, and other areas of Asia, as well as Africa, where the traditional diet is high in carbohydrates, insulin resistance and diabetes are uncommon because people are very active and obesity is rare.

"About a quarter of insulin resistance is caused by obesity, and another quarter is related to how physically active you are. The other half is genetic," says Reaven. Whether you eat a high-carbohydrate or low-carbohydrate diet won't affect your likelihood of becoming insulin resistant. And if you are insulin resistant, you can lose weight and reduce insulin resistance on a high- or a low-carbohydrate diet, as long as calories are low.

Losing weight often has dramatic results. "Once insulin-resistant individuals control calories, start exercising, and lose weight, their insulin resistance often disappears," says Reaven. "Losing as little as 10 pounds can be enough to reverse insulin resistance."

WHAT ABOUT THE GLYCEMIC INDEX?

Recent diet books don't just warn us about the insulin response and the calories from carbohydrates. They tell us that we need to be concerned with the *rate* at which the carbohydrate-rich foods increase blood sugar. The scientific tool to measure this blood sugar rise is called the glycemic index. The theory is that high-glycemic foods, which cause a rapid rise in blood sugar, are more likely to increase body fat than low-glycemic-index foods.

We know that pure sugar causes blood sugar to rise quickly. But white bread is even quicker. Many dietary staples have a high glycemic index: pasta, rice, bread, breakfast cereals, potatoes, corn, beets, even carrots. Other low-glycemic-index foods, like dry beans, nuts, and dairy foods, cause a slower, more sustained blood sugar rise.

The glycemic index is a poor guide for food selection, either for nutrition or for weight management. The main reason is that there's little correlation between an individual food's glycemic index and that of a whole meal or dietary pattern. We know that dietary patterns that have a low glycemic index are linked with lower risk of diabetes and perhaps other diseases. But that doesn't mean that low-glycemic-index foods like ice cream are "good," or high-glycemic-index foods like carrots are "bad." "Once you start putting together meals, there are just too many variables, including the way foods are digested, metabolized, assimilated, and absorbed," says Reaven. As states University of California at Davis nutrition professor Judith Stern, "The glycemic index comes into play if you're eating a single food. But we don't do that. We eat mixed diets." Even if it were more reliable, the glycemic index wouldn't help you lose weight or keep it off. "There is zero evidence that the glycemic index affects weight," says Reaven.

Some studies do suggest that the glycemic response to foods affects hunger and satiety. It's a reasonable hypothesis. We know that blood sugar (glucose) affects hunger and satiety. When blood sugar declines rapidly, you feel hungry and eat; when blood sugar rises, people eat less. Our bodies monitor glucose closely, because it's essential for all cells, and is the only fuel our brains can use. There are glucose-sensitive cells in the brain, liver, and perhaps the gut that monitor the rate at which glucose is being used. The results from satiety studies, though, are conflicting. Some studies find that high-glycemic foods are *more* satiating than low-glycemic foods, while other studies find they are *less* satiating. It's not yet clear whether the most satiating effect occurs when you get a quick blood sugar rise (high-glycemic foods) or a slow sustained release of blood sugar, which keeps satiety signals around longer (low-glycemic foods).

Although the glycemic index has been promoted as a guide for foods that help to control hunger and body weight, scientific evidence for this approach is slim. If you follow the glycemic index for your food choices, you will be avoiding many nutritious foods, including some that are low in energy density and high in fiber. Yet those are the foods you should be selecting.

THE CASE FOR FIBER

The first diet book I (Barbara) remember as a blockbuster was *The F-Plan Diet* by Audrey Eyton. It was 1982, I was living in Britain, and the book took Europe by storm. The premise: A high-fiber diet fills you up by adding bulk to food without calories, decreases the digestion of the calories you eat along with it, and gives you sensory satisfaction because high-fiber foods require a lot of chewing. "The

How Much Fiber Is in Your Diet?

How much fiber do you consume? Here's a quick method to estimate your daily fiber intake. For each food category below, list the number of servings you eat daily. Then multiply the number of servings by the fiber content and add up the numbers. This total gives a rough estimate of your daily fiber intake in grams. For a more accurate measure, refer to "The Fiber Content of Foods," p. 65, and the nutrition labels on foods.

Food	Daily Servings	Fiber Content per Serving	Fiber Intake (grams)
Breakfast Cereals	*	*	= _____
Whole Grains	One serving = 1 slice whole-wheat bread, 1 small whole-wheat roll, ½ cup brown rice or whole-grain pasta	2.5	= _____
Refined Grains	One serving = 1 slice white bread, 1 small white roll, ½ English muffin, ½ cup white rice or pasta	1.0	= _____
Vegetables	One serving = ½ cup vegetables, 2 cups leafy greens, ¾ cup vegetable juice	2.0	= _____
Legumes	One serving = ½ cup cooked kidney or black beans, lentils, or split peas	6.0	= _____
Fruit	One serving = 1 medium-sized fruit, half a grapefruit, ½ cup berries, or ¼ cup dried fruit	2.0	= _____

* refer to "Breakfast Cereals of 200 Calories," p. 177, or nutrition label

TOTAL = _____

slimming benefits of the F-Plan Diet start in the mouth, continue in the stomach, extend to the blood, and reach a grand finale with that final flush," wrote Eyton.

It was that final flush and rumblings in the gut that dampened the enthusiasm of many who tried this diet. If you start eating a lot more high-fiber foods, you can feel bloated and get gas. When you increase the fiber in your diet, you should do so gradually, over several weeks, to avoid flatulence and other gastrointestinal side effects of a too-rapid increase.

Fiber intake has been linked with slimness since the early seventies, when studies in Africa found that obesity was rare in rural areas where the traditional plant-based diet was exceptionally rich in fiber. While Americans average about 15 grams of fiber daily, many rural Africans take in 80 grams. Even a modest increase in fiber may be linked with lower body weight. In England, lean adults averaged 19 grams a day while obese ones consumed only 13. Vegetarians, who tend to eat a high-fiber diet because fiber is found only in plant foods, are leaner on average than meat eaters.

Can fiber help you stay full on fewer calories? Yes, modestly. It reduces the energy density of foods, increases satiety, and may reduce the body's absorption of calories. The effect of fiber on the energy density of foods, however, is modest compared to the effect of water in foods. Even if you increase your daily fiber intake from 10 to 30 grams a day, that's less than an ounce. Have a cup of low-fat broth-based soup before lunch, by contrast, and you're consuming an extra 8 ounces, most of it water.

But fiber appears to increase satiety through other mechanisms, too. Fiber-rich foods take a lot of chewing, providing sensory experience that contributes to satiety. Fiber also slows the passage of food through the digestive system, so satiety signals are stimulated for longer.

Consuming more fiber is particularly useful in hunger control when you are keeping calories low, that is, when you're trying to lose weight. Both soluble and insoluble fiber increase satiety and help with weight loss when added as a supplement in a drink, or better yet, when people simply eat more high-fiber bread, fruits, vegetables, and breakfast cereals, research shows.

Consider fiber when you make food choices. Do you choose juice or a whole piece of fruit, which has more fiber? Do you eat your baked potato, cucumber, or apple with the peel? When you choose grain products, do you look for higher-fiber versions?

Fiber Content of Foods

To consume more fiber, eat more whole fruits and vegetables, whole grains, and beans. Nuts are also rich in fiber, but they are energy dense, so eat them in small amounts. Use the following list to guide your food choices. It is adapted from research conducted by the Tufts University School of Medicine in Boston and published in the *Tufts Health & Nutrition Letter*. (For fiber information on breakfast cereals, an important source, see "Breakfast Cereals of 200 Calories," p. 177.)

Fruits*	Grams of Fiber
Apple (with skin)	4
Banana	3
Blueberries, ½ cup	2
Cantaloupe, 1 cup diced	1
Dates, ⅛ cup dry, chopped	2
Grapefruit, ½	2
Grapes, 1 cup	2
Nectarine (with skin)	2
Orange	3
Peach (with skin)	2
Pear (with skin)	4
Plum (with skin)	1
Prunes (dried), 10	2
Raisins, ⅛ cup	1
Raspberries, ½ cup	4
Strawberries, ½ cup	2
Watermelon, 1 cup diced	1

*All values are for 1 medium-size fruit unless otherwise indicated.

Vegetables†	Grams of Fiber
Broccoli, ½ cup cooked, chopped	2
Broccoli, ½ cup chopped	1
Brussels sprouts, ½ cup cooked	3
Carrot, 1 medium	2
Carrots, ½ cup cooked	3
Cauliflower, ½ cup cooked	2
Celery, 1 stalk	1
Corn, ½ cup cooked	2

Cucumber, ½ cup sliced	0.5
French fries, 1 small (2.5 ounces)serving	2
Green beans, ½ cup cooked (frozen)	2
Iceberg lettuce, 1 cup shredded	1
Peas, ½ cup cooked (frozen)	4
Peppers, ½ cup chopped	1
Potato, baked, with skin	5
Potato, baked, without skin	2
Potato, ½ cup mashed	2
Romaine lettuce, 1 cup shredded	1
Spinach, ½ cup chopped	1
Spinach, ½ cup cooked (frozen)	3
Sweet potato, baked with skin	3
Tomato, 1 medium	1

†All values are for raw, uncooked vegetables unless otherwise indicated.

Grains, Legumes (Beans**, Chickpeas, Lentils, Lima Beans), and Nuts	Grams of Fiber
Black beans, ½ cup	8
Bread, 1 slice, white	1
Bread, 1 slice, whole-wheat	2
Bran muffin, 1 medium	3
Chickpeas, ½ cup	5
Kidney beans, ½ cup	7
Lentils, ½ cup	8
Lima beans, ½ cup	6
Oatmeal, 1 cup cooked	4
Pasta, ½ cup cooked	1
Peanuts, ½ cup	6
Peanut butter, 2 tablespoons, chunky	2
Popcorn, 3 cups air-popped	2
Rice, 1 cup cooked, white	1
Rice, 1 cup cooked, brown	2
Sesame seeds, 2 tablespoons	1
Sunflower seeds, ⅛ cup	2
Tortilla chips, 1 cup (1.5 oz)	1
Walnuts, ¼ cup chopped	2
Wheat germ, ¼ cup	4

**Values are for canned or cooked beans.

BREAKFAST BENEFITS

It's ironic that breakfast is the meal most often skipped by dieters. People who skip breakfast end up eating more calories because they make up for the skipped breakfast later in the day when they are surrounded by energy-dense convenience foods. Skipping breakfast also slows the rate at which you burn calories. The reason is that metabolism slows while we sleep, while the process of digesting food revs it up again. If you don't eat breakfast, your metabolism may stay slower throughout the morning.

Leaner people are less likely to skip breakfast than obese people. If you're on a weight loss diet, eating breakfast will improve your success. At Vanderbilt University in Nashville, fifty-two obese women, who usually skipped breakfast, were asked to include that morning meal for 3 months. As a result, they had more control over their eating, consumed less fat, and lost more weight than a control group that continued to skip breakfast.

For many people, breakfast is the easiest meal at which to increase fiber intake because it is easy to include whole-grain products and fruits. Extra fiber at breakfast, in turn, can help you eat less at lunch and for the rest of the day. In Minneapolis, volunteers who ate high-fiber cereals ate fewer calories at breakfast *and* fewer calories at lunch, saving about 150 calories for the day.

The best choice is a high-fiber cereal with low-fat (1 percent) or skim milk and fruit. People who eat ready-to-eat cereal consume more iron, more calcium, more folate, and more fiber than people who eat other breakfasts. It's not just the cereal but the company it keeps: calcium-rich milk and fruit, often a good source of fiber, folate, and vitamins C and A. Starting your morning this way has also been shown in a number of studies to be associated with reduced hunger and food intake later in the day.

THE *VOLUMETRICS* OF GRAINS, VEGETABLES, AND FRUITS

There is one dietary action that will both increase your fiber intake and dramatically lower the energy density of your diet: Increase the

160 Calories of Breakfast Cereal

It's breakfast time. Your cereal is ready. But how much can you eat? That depends on several factors: fat, fiber, sugar, and shape. These are the figures without milk:

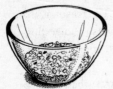

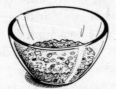

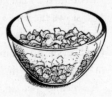

Regular granola. E.D.: 4.6. Serving size: ⅓ cup. This high-fat, high-sugar cereal packs down tightly, so you get only a puny serving.

Low-fat granola. E.D.: 3.9. Serving size: just under ½ cup. Just cutting fat helps a little, but it's still a pretty small amount.

Frosted flakes. E.D.: 4.0. Serving size: 1 cup. Flakes, even sugary ones, create more volume, so even though the energy density hasn't gone down, you get more in a bowl.

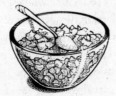

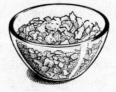

Wheat flakes with 1 teaspoon sugar. E.D.: 3.7. Serving size: 1⅓ cups. When you bring the sugar down by purchasing regular flakes and adding a small amount of sugar yourself, you can eat more.

Bran flakes. E.D.: 3.3. Serving size: 1⅔ cups. The most Volumetric choice of all: low in fat, high in fiber, made of volume-boosting flakes. If you add a teaspoon of sugar, you can keep the calories the same by eating 1½ cups of cereal. Or use a sugar substitute.

amount and variety of vegetables and fruits. These carbohydrate-containing foods are truly extraordinary. You can eat virtually as much as you want of many of these, and you'll wind up consuming fewer calories. In Roland Weinsier's weight loss program at the University of Alabama at Birmingham, even people on low-calorie weight loss diets (1,200 calories a day) may eat as many vegetables (cooked without added fat) and whole fruits as they want. They practice portion control over more energy-dense choices such as dried fruits; starchy vegetables like potatoes, lima beans, and corn; breads and grains; meats; and dairy foods; but not for whole fruits and vegetables. Says Weinsier, "These displace more energy-dense foods. Unless you force yourself to eat an enormous quantity, when you eat lots of fruits and vegetables, your calorie intake goes down."

A 400-Calorie Spaghetti Dinner

Just how much can vegetables increase your portion size at dinner? A lot! Check out the difference between a high-fat, low-vegetable dish and a low-fat, high-vegetable dish below: With less fat and plenty of added vegetables, energy density drops by more than half:

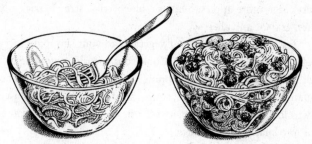

Spaghetti Alfredo (left). Ingredients: 1 cup cooked spaghetti, ½ cup Alfredo sauce. E.D.: 1.5. Serving size: 1½ cups.

Spaghetti primavera (right). Ingredients: 1 cup cooked spaghetti, ¾ cup canned tomatoes, ¾ cup cooked summer squash, ½ cup cooked mushrooms, 1 cup cooked broccoli, 2 teaspoons olive oil, basil, oregano, 2 teaspoons Parmesan cheese. E.D.: 0.6. Serving size: 3½ cups.

Increasing the variety of vegetables you eat is a relatively simple way to lower calories. For most of us there's plenty of room for improvement: Half of all the vegetables that Americans eat are fresh and frozen potatoes (often fried), lettuce, processed tomatoes, and onions. People think that fruits and vegetables need to be raw for maximum health benefits, but they can be frozen, canned, or dried and still have as good nutritional quality. Says Elizabeth Pivonka, president of the Produce for Better Health Foundation, "If you make pasta primavera with 2 cups of vegetables and a half-cup of pasta, instead of 2 cups of pasta and a half-cup of vegetables, you cut calories in half."

Make it a point to find more fruits and vegetables you like and include them in your meals. If you don't like a particular vegetable, that's fine. Skip it. But seek others. Every day, try to include at least one dark green or yellow fruit or vegetable, such as green or red leaf lettuce, mixed baby greens, spinach, squash, peppers, apricots, peaches, mangos, cantaloupe. Enjoy citrus fruit (orange, grapefruit, tangerine) every day. A few times a week, eat a nutritious and cancer-protective "cruciferous" vegetable such as broccoli, cauliflower, Brussels sprouts, or red and green cabbage. Cook with onions and garlic. Have tomatoes, either raw or cooked into sauce, a few times a week. Eat more apples, bananas, blueberries, strawberries, plums, pears, grapes, and cherries.

Try adding a new fruit or vegetable to your shopping cart this week. Next week, try another. Cook your favorite vegetable differently, perhaps with a new seasoning. Adding vegetables to dishes you already like, like omelets, soups, stir-fries, and stews, is an easy way to lower the energy density of your diet. So is incorporating fruit into snacks and desserts.

EASY WAYS TO GET MORE FRUITS AND VEGETABLES INTO YOUR DIET

Here are some ways to get more fruits and vegetables into your life:

- Add fruit to breakfast cereal.

- Add grapes and sliced apples to chicken salad, or tomatoes, radishes, and bell peppers to a tuna salad.

- Top broiled chicken or fish with salsa.

- Stock your kitchen with fruits and vegetables that keep well, such as onions, garlic, potatoes, squash, carrots, apples, oranges, and bananas. Then you can pick up more perishable items like lettuce or green vegetables on the way home.

- Get vegetable plastic bags. They have tiny holes that let produce stay fresh longer. Or simply take plastic food bags and make several tiny punctures with a fork.

- For convenience, buy ready-to-eat bagged veggies or veggies from the salad bar. Put them on a plate with nonfat ranch dressing, and munch on them while you're making dinner—instead of reaching for cheese or chips.

- Pack bite-size fruit or veggies in lunch bags for school or work: small apples, seedless grapes, mini bananas, berries, orange quarters, cherry tomatoes, baby carrots, snow peas, green beans.

- Add fresh fruits and vegetables to dishes you like: berries or bananas to yogurt; vegetables to pasta and pizza; tomatoes, onions, grated carrots, and dark green lettuces like Romaine to sandwiches; fresh or frozen veggies to canned soup.

- At your next barbecue, put vegetables on one skewer, fruit on another.

- At parties, serve raw veggies with salsa, and on another plate, fruit wedges with nonfat yogurt dip.

- Learn to love your microwave. Fresh asparagus, washed with a little water still dripping off it, and a squeeze of lemon or a teaspoon of balsamic vinegar, in a covered microwave-safe dish, takes only 2 or 3 minutes on high power.

Speaking of dessert, what about sugar? Sugar may have brought more pleasure to humankind than any other single dietary substance, yet it evokes mixed emotions. We like it, but we feel guilty about eating it. We're afraid it's bad for us, that it makes us gain weight and rots our teeth. Our ambivalence has historical roots: Since sugar was introduced into Europe in the late Middle Ages, it has been considered a medicine of an almost divine purity—and a wicked threat to health.

At the moment, the pendulum has turned against sugar once again, with popular diet books telling us that sugar causes obesity by raising insulin levels. By now, you know that these theories relating insulin and glycemic index to weight loss have not been proven. Sugar does have a high glycemic index, but as long as you control calories, the amount of sugar in your diet makes no difference for weight loss. At Duke University, overweight women on a 1,100-calorie weight loss diet lost as much weight on a diet that got 43 percent of its calories from sugar as on one that got only 4 percent of its calories from sugar!

Yet sugars may still affect obesity if they entice us into consuming more calories than we need. Sweet foods are easy to overeat, but this is not because sugars sneak in unnoticed by satiety systems. Sugars and starch, and even fat, have similar effects on satiety. The main reason we overeat sugars is taste. Humans are born with a sweet tooth. Even in the cozy comfort of the uterus, the fetus swallows amniotic fluid, which contains sugars. Since the taste system starts to function in the womb, it is likely that the sweet taste is first experienced there. Within hours of birth, a baby prefers sweet tastes. This encourages feeding on breast milk, which is rich in milk sugar (lactose). A sweet tooth stays with people into adulthood. It varies, to be sure. People are born with a certain preference for sweetness, and whether they eat lots of sugary foods or few doesn't affect this preference. As people age, though, the sweet tooth eventually declines. It is most intense in childhood, adolescence, and early adulthood.

The main concern with sugars is that they can encourage consumption of too many calories. This is particularly true for foods that combine fat and sugars, such as chocolate, cookies, candy bars, and cakes, which are both delicious and highly energy-dense. Some researchers have found that sugar/fat combinations stimulate the brain's pleasure centers, increasing the production of endorphins, the body's "feel good" chemicals. No wonder they are hard to resist!

Sugars can contribute plenty of calories even when they're not paired with fat. Sugars are moderately high in energy density, with 4 calories per gram. Many low-fat, high-sugar confections or cookies are so low in water content that they contain nearly as many calories per portion as the high-fat versions they replace.

The U.S. Department of Agriculture's Dietary Guidelines tell us to choose a diet moderate in added sugars. They suggest that added sugars—those not naturally occurring in foods—should be no more than 10 percent of our total calories. The USDA recommends these limits for added sugars: 6 teaspoons for a caloric intake of 1,600 calories, 12 for 2,200 calories, and 18 for 2,800 calories. A typical 12-ounce can of soda pop has about 10 teaspoons worth of sugars. It's *added* sugars that have been a concern, since naturally occurring sugars are found primarily in foods that we are being encouraged to eat such as fruits, vegetables, and low-fat milk and dairy foods. A medium banana, with about 4 teaspoons of sugars, is a good source of fiber, potassium, and vitamin C, and, like most fruits, has lots of water. So its energy density is less than 1 calorie per gram. The energy density of pure sugar, as we've noted, is 4.

Is your intake of added sugars too high? Some people are clearly taking too much. It's easy to do. A teaspoon of sugar contains around 16 calories. Suppose you are on a 1,600-calorie-a-day diet. If you drink one sweet drink with 10 teaspoons of sugar, or 160 calories, that's your 10 percent added sugars for the day. It can add up quickly in other foods as well. If you cut out 160 calories from sugars a day, and don't replace them with other calories, you'll lose an extra pound every 3 weeks.

You needn't banish sugars. They are neither villains nor heroes. Too much can surely throw a diet out of balance, but moderate amounts can make nutritious eating a little more fun. One way to satisfy a preference for sweetness without adding pounds to our bodies is to emphasize naturally sweet foods low in energy density, like fruit ices and fruit-based desserts. Another is the judicious use of sugars to make other low-energy-dense foods taste better, such as a teaspoon of sugar on cereal. If you make a baked apple with a tablespoon of sugar, you'll still be eating a dessert with a low energy density. It will taste sweet and delicious, and it will fill you up.

SUGAR SUBSTITUTES

Another way to enjoy the sweet taste while controlling calories is to choose foods or drinks made with sugar substitutes. They can help you cut calories and control hunger, and provide you with a wider variety of low-energy-dense food choices. According to the scientific evidence, they are also safe. "Aspartame, acesulfame K, sucralose, and saccharin are nontoxic," says Drexell University food science professor Stanley Segall. "Artificially sweetened foods, used in moderation, pose no health risk."

One myth has been that sugar substitutes stimulate hunger. We and other researchers have demonstrated that this simply isn't true. When used instead of sugar in foods, sugar substitutes help to reduce hunger and food intake. In certain sweet foods, sugar substitutes can substantially lower the energy density and increase the amount you can eat. Consider nonfat flavored yogurt. For 80 calories you can have ½ cup yogurt sweetened with sugar or ¾ cup of the same yogurt sweetened with aspartame:

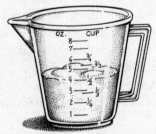

Nonfat flavored yogurt sweetened with sugar. E.D.: 0.7. Serving size: ½ cup.

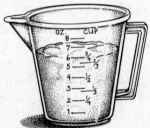

Nonfat flavored yogurt sweetened with aspartame. E.D.: 0.5. Serving size: ¾ cup.

You've substantially reduced the energy density of your dessert, so you can eat a reasonable portion. To make this work, though, you really have to *replace* a sugary food with a food sweetened with a sugar substitute.

If you use sugar substitutes as a part of a planned program to lose weight and keep it off, they can be useful. At Harvard University, obese women in a 19-week weight loss program who were encouraged to use aspartame-sweetened products lost the same amount of weight as women who used sugar. But the women in the aspartame group liked the diet better, and 3 years later, they had kept off half the weight they had lost, while the women in the other group had regained all their lost weight.

As part of an integrated plan to reduce the energy density of your diet, sugar substitutes can make meals and snacks more varied and pleasant. But they are only one part of your strategy, and they won't help if you simply eat more. People can play mind games with food. If you order a diet cola to go with your cheeseburger and large fries, the diet drink won't magically eliminate the calories from the burger and fries!

SUMMARY

- Enjoy your staple foods—bread, pasta, potatoes, rice. These complex carbohydrates are the core of a healthful, weight management diet.

- Carbohydrates should make up about 55 percent of your calories. Most of these calories should come from complex carbohydrates, rich in starch and fiber. Emphasize those low in energy density to enhance satiety.

- Neither insulin resistance nor eating foods with a high glycemic index leads to weight gain. If you are overweight and sedentary, however, you may be insulin resistant; to lower your health risks, cut calories, lose weight, and increase physical activity.

- Aim to consume 20–30 grams of fiber a day. Increase your fiber intake gradually by eating more high-fiber cereal, whole grains,

legumes, vegetables, and fruits. This can help you to feel full
and to eat less if you are trying to reduce your calorie intake.

- Eat a minimum of 2 servings of fruit and 3 servings of vegetables, every day. Whole fresh fruit and vegetables cooked without added fat are so low in energy density that you can eat
  satisfying portions, even on a calorie-controlled diet.

- Use added sugars in moderation to make nutritious foods of low
  energy density more enjoyable. If you eat energy-dense sweets or
  foods that combine sugars and fat, keep portions small.

- Sugar substitutes, as part of your program to lower the energy
  density of your diet, can help you to feel full on fewer calories.

Protein

Meat is a natural nourishment of man because his
stomach is too small to deal with the bulk of food
he would have to consume if his diet were restricted
to fruit and vegetables.
— JEAN-ANTHELME BRILLAT-SAVARIN,
La Physiologie du gout, 1825

IN THE REBELLION AGAINST LOW-FAT diets, protein is the new
king. Diet books tell you that you can lose weight by eating more
high-fat meat and cheese. They say more protein keeps you meta-
bolically fit. Protein does have a role in weight management, but
not for the reasons you may have read. They have overlooked what
could be the biggest advantage for weight management:
High-protein foods can decrease hunger and prolong satiety
more than foods high in either carbohydrate or fat.
Because the high-protein diets that are in vogue restrict food
choices, they are actually low-calorie diets in disguise. By emphasiz-

ing protein foods, they can help people feel less hungry while greatly restricting calories. You can lose weight this way, but you won't learn eating habits that will keep the weight off. That's because standard high-protein American fare like cheeseburgers is high in energy density. You have to restrict portions to cut calories. Once you eat normal portions again, you'll consume too many calories and regain the weight.

We've got two better suggestions:

- *Maintain your daily protein intake at the recommended level, whether you are trying to lose weight or keep weight off.* Your protein needs stay the same whatever your calorie level and depend on how much you weigh. To calculate your protein level, see "How Much Protein Do You Need?" (p. 81).

- *Emphasize low-energy-dense protein sources.* Choose moderate portions of *lean* protein-rich beef, chicken, seafood, low-fat dairy foods, and legumes, which are fairly low in energy density, and combine them with low-energy-dense grains, vegetables, and fruits. That way, you'll lower the energy density of your entire dietary pattern, which will allow you to find a permanent way of eating that lets you stay full on fewer calories.

Eating enough protein-rich foods of low energy density is a good strategy for increasing satiety, especially if you are trying to lose weight. But eating more protein than your body needs is not going to boost your metabolism, build more muscle, or make you thinner!

PROTEIN HELPS YOU FEEL FULL

The enhanced satiety associated with eating protein was first noted in 1955, when people on low-calorie diets, who ate enough protein, reported feeling satiated. When protein intake fell, they felt hungry all the time.

Since then, the "protein satiety effect" has been repeatedly demonstrated. Studies in Scotland, Denmark, Sweden, and England showed that eating a high-protein breakfast or lunch was associated

What Is Protein?

Proteins are chains of complex molecules called amino acids. When we consume a food that contains protein, our bodies break it down into individual amino acids, which are then re-formed into many different proteins we need to function, including enzymes, hormones, and antibodies. Our bodies need protein every day to replace body proteins that normally break down and need to be rebuilt. If we consume protein in excess of our need for amino acids, it is converted into sugars and burned as fuel, or stored as body fat.

with decreased hunger and lower food intake at the next meal. And when Canadian men were given either high-protein or moderate-protein meals for 6 days, and could eat as much as they liked, those eating more protein took in fewer calories each day. Concludes Lavalle University nutrition professor Angelo Tremblay, "A high-protein diet produces satiety with fewer calories."

Psychology may play a part in the satiety effect. We think of meals as more complete or substantial if they contain meat or other high-protein entrees. Are certain kinds of protein more satiating than others? One study did find that different types of meat affect satiety differently. They compared a meal with the same amount of protein from beef, chicken, or fish. Over the next 3 hours, the researchers found, one protein source consistently yielded a greater sense of fullness: fish.

Protein can also affect the rate at which you burn calories. The body is very inefficient at converting excess protein calories to body fat. We can do it, but we lose about 40 percent of excess protein calories in the process. "You create more carbon dioxide," explains protein expert Peter Reeds of Baylor College of Medicine in Houston. "Essentially, you're blowing excess protein off as heat."

WHY HIGH-PROTEIN DIETS ARE UNSUSTAINABLE

Enhanced satiety and burning calories off as heat are benefits for dieters. But it is almost impossible to stay on a high-protein diet for long. The way metabolism increases to burn excess protein hints at the reason: Our bodies regulate protein carefully. If you take in too little, your body conserves it. If you take in too much, your body burns it.

Populations all around the world consume 10–15 percent of

Is Too Much Protein Unhealthy?

Most American adults consume more protein than they need. Is that unhealthy?

There's little evidence that it is. Even at twice the recommended amounts, our bodies are good at ridding themselves of excess protein. It strains the kidneys, but that is a health concern primarily for infants, and for adults with kidney failure or diabetes. Excess protein, especially from animal flesh, also causes the body to excrete extra calcium, which could increase osteoporosis risk, but only in people who don't consume adequate calcium and vitamin D.

High-protein, low-calorie diets don't pose an immediate health risk. The exception: those that also restrict carbohydrates to such low levels that they create a metabolic state that can stress the kidneys and cause the body to break down muscle.

The real health risk comes when you stop the diet. If you scale up to a normal calorie level, but continue eating mostly animal sources of protein, like steaks and burgers, with too few fruits and vegetables, you'll increase your risk of heart disease, diabetes, and certain kinds of cancers. "People who eat a lot of meat tend to have high-fat, high-saturated fat diets *and* low intakes of fruits and vegetables," says University of Colorado School of Medicine professor Tim Byers. "Yet the one thing we can conclude safely is that people who eat a substantial proportion of their foods from fruits, vegetables, and whole grains have less heart disease and cancer."

---

calories from protein, not the 30 percent recommended by some diet books. This 10–15 percent level of protein is found over a remarkably diverse set of cultures, wherever people have access to an adequate diet. Our bodies have mechanisms, such as amino acid receptors in the gut, that help us sense how much protein we are consuming. Says Reeds, "I believe that human beings regulate protein intake."

Surveys have not found an association between protein intake and leanness. Lean people don't consume more protein than overweight people. When researchers have found a link between protein intake and body weight, being overweight was associated with higher protein intake! This is probably because high-fat meats are often the most preferred foods of overweight men. That may help explain the popularity of high-protein diets in men. But eating a high-protein diet, whether it is one based on meats, eggs and dairy products, or one of the high-protein liquid diets, is not a sustainable weight management strategy. As we saw with Oprah Winfrey, who adopted a high-protein liquid diet in the eighties, it's possible to lose weight on high-protein diets, but the weight returns with a vengeance when the diet stops. These diets do not teach eating habits that help you manage calories when you are surrounded by a variety of tasty, energy-dense foods.

WEIGHT LOSS THAT LASTS

How can you use the satiating power of protein to your advantage? The answer is simple: Maintain your protein intake at the level recommended for your body weight. This is good advice both when you are losing weight and when you are working to keep it off:

- **Weight loss.** When you cut calories, don't eat more high-protein foods than you usually do—but don't eat fewer. Cut calories by choosing normal portions of lean protein sources like lean beef, chicken, seafood, beans, skim milk, and low-fat dairy, by eating fewer high-fat foods, by eating smaller portions of energy-dense high-carbohydrate snacks, by watching bread portions, and by emphasizing whole grains, vegetables, and fruits. Cut calories from fat and from excess carbohydrates, not from protein. Why? It's not just the enhanced satiety and calorie burning. When you lose weight, you lose not just body fat, but also muscle. Yet muscle keeps metabolism high, which helps prevent weight regain. Maintaining adequate protein intake during weight loss will minimize muscle loss.

- **Weight Maintenance.** It's only when you cut calories well below what's needed to maintain body weight that you are at risk of consuming too little protein. When you are eating enough food and calories to maintain your new lower body weight, you'll consume enough protein. The American diet, whether a carnivore's delight or a vegetarian paradise, is so

How Much Protein Do You Need?

The amount of protein you need each day is based on how much you weigh: 0.4 grams per pound of body weight. Most people get more than enough.

If You Weigh This Many Pounds ...	You'll Need About This many Grams of Protein
110	40
130	47
150	54
180	65
210	76

It's easy to satisfy these protein requirements. You'll get more than enough if you eat 2–3 servings a day from protein-rich foods such as meat, poultry, eggs, seafood, and beans. Dairy foods are also good sources.

Food	Serving Size	Protein (grams)	Calories	Energy Density
Egg, boiled	1	6	78	1.5
Sirloin steak	3 ounces	26	315	1.8
Ground beef patty, lean, broiled	3 ounces	21	230	2.7
Chicken breast, without skin, roasted	3 ounces	26	140	1.7
Tuna, canned, water-packed	3 ounces	20	110	1.3
Pork chop, lean, grilled	3 ounces	26	172	2.0
Black beans	½ cup	7	110	0.9
Chickpeas	½ cup	7	134	1.6
Milk, whole	1 cup (8 ounces)	8	150	0.6
Milk, skim	1 cup (8 ounces)	8	86	0.35
Yogurt, low-fat, fruit	1 cup (8 ounces)	12	240	1.0
Cheddar cheese	1 ounce	7	115	4.0

rich in protein that if calories are adequate, protein intake will be adequate. After your weight loss phase, continue eating normal portions of lean protein foods, and increase calories by eating more foods rich in complex carbohydrates of low energy density.

Whether you are losing weight or keeping it off, make sure there is a good source of low-fat protein at most meals. It could be skim milk with your cereal, water-packed tuna for lunch, or a lean piece of steak for dinner. It needn't be every meal. You may also want to find some high-protein snacks that you enjoy: yogurt, lean turkey slices, leftover kabobs, or black bean dip served with veggies.

Let energy density guide your choices. Low-fat red meats such as lean ham steak or sirloin steak give you more to eat than even a "lean" hamburger. Poultry without the skin, such as roasted turkey breast, is lower in energy density still, while lean fish, such as baked perch, gives you the most satisfying portion of all, as these illustrations of 150-calorie portions demonstrate.

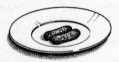

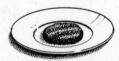

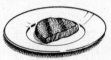

Italian pork sausage. E.D.: 3.2. Serving size: 1.7 ounces.

Hamburger made with lean ground beef, broiled. E.D.: 2.7. Serving size: 2 ounces.

Lean sirloin steak, broiled. E.D.: 1.9. Serving size: 2.9 ounces.

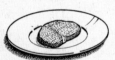

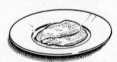

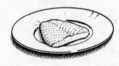

Lean ham* (11 percent fat). E.D.: 1.8. Serving size: 2.9 ounces.

Turkey breast, roasted without skin. E.D.: 1.3. Serving size: 3.9 ounces.

Perch, baked. E.D.: 1.1. Serving size: 4.8 ounces.

Choose lean protein foods (fish, turkey, very lean ham or steak) to eat more satisfying portions.

* *If you choose extra lean ham (4 percent fat), your serving size would be 4.1 ounces.*

Be wary of energy-dense high-protein snacks. One recent weight loss book advocating a high-protein diet, for example, recommends snacks such as sunflower seeds, walnuts, macadamia nuts, peanuts, pork rinds, meat and cheese on crackers, peanut butter crackers, and beef jerky. These are all high in energy density and very easy to overeat! You get such small portions that regardless of the protein content, you will feel hungry.

Use the principles of *Volumetrics* to boost the satisfaction you'll get from a portion of meat. Two or 3 ounces (a standard "serving size") of beef, pork, chicken, or fish may seem a forlorn presence on your plate. But slice your steak into small strips and stir-fry it in a nonstick pan with a large amount of vegetables and you'll get a nice hefty portion that's still fairly low in total calories. When you combine protein's satiating power with the core energy-density principles of this book, you get a really satisfying meal.

SUMMARY

- Protein-rich foods are particularly satiating. They can help to control hunger when calories are restricted and may help you lose weight in the short term. But once you start eating normally again, high-protein foods like high-fat meats and dairy products are often high in energy density, so you'll regain the weight.

- When you are losing weight, maintain adequate amounts of protein-rich foods, but cut calories and energy density by choosing lean protein sources.

- To maintain weight loss and prevent weight gain, continue eating the recommended level of protein for your body weight. Increase calories to your maintenance level by eating more complex carbohydrates low in energy density.

- To lose weight and keep it off, choose high-protein foods of low energy density and cooked with little added fat, such as lean steak, pork tenderloin, chicken or turkey breast, fish, shellfish, egg-white omelets, beans, and tofu.

Alcohol

*It was my Uncle George who discovered that alcohol was
food well in advance of modern medical thought.*
— P. G. WODEHOUSE,
The Inimitable Jeeves, 1923

IF YOU DRINK ALCOHOLIC BEVERAGES, you may wonder how
they affect your weight. So do scientists. It's a hot topic, and the
answers matter for weight management: The average American
adult who drinks moderately consumes 5–10 percent of his or her
calories as alcohol. ("Moderate" is defined as up to 1 alcoholic
drink a day for a woman, 2 for a man.)

Population studies find no link between alcohol consumption
and body weight. In women, those who drink actually weigh less
than those who don't. Yet careful research on metabolism and eating and drinking behavior reveals that alcoholic beverages do pose
a challenge for many people trying to control calories. Certain patterns of alcohol and food consumption are particularly likely to
promote weight gain. Consider:

- Alcohol is energy dense. A gram of alcohol has 7 calories, compared to 4 for carbohydrate or protein. An ounce of pure alcohol has 200 calories, and mixed drinks often contain more.

- Our bodies metabolize alcohol in ways that enhance the likelihood that excess calories will wind up as body fat.

- Calories from alcoholic beverages can slink into our bodies
  without triggering satiety signals, so we don't compensate by
  eating less.

Don't fret: We're not going to tell you to stop drinking to lose
weight. If you'd like to try it for a few weeks, to see if it jump-starts
your weight loss efforts, that's fine. But we want to give you options
that will work for the long term, and if you drink moderately now,

abstaining is unlikely to become a long-term choice. Nor does it need to be. Moderate drinking is consistent with weight management and has health benefits for many adults.

But certain drinking patterns can make it harder to control calories. We'll tell you what those patterns are, so you can try to change them.

WHERE DO ALCOHOL CALORIES GO?

After a drink, you may feel flushed. Is that your metabolism getting revved up? Are you burning up extra calories? Unfortunately, for moderate drinkers the answer is no. Alcohol doesn't cause the body to burn calories any faster or slower than any other nutrient. That's the conclusion of several metabolic studies, including those performed at the Dunn Clinical Nutrition Centre in Cambridge, England. Healthy young men ate a high-fat lunch in a "whole-body calorimeter," a room that measures calories burned by gauging oxygen use. On some days, the men got 80-proof Calvados brandy as a substitute for some of the lunch's carbohydrate, while on other days the brandy's calories were simply added to the lunch's calories.

When calories remained the same, alcohol had no effect on metabolism. The men metabolized their lunches with alcohol as efficiently as their lunches without alcohol. But when alcohol was *added* on top of the high-fat, high-calorie meal, less dietary fat was burned and more was stored as body fat. The reason is that the body gives preference to getting rid of alcohol, a poison that can't be stored. Your body breaks down alcohol faster than carbohydrates, carbohydrates faster than protein, and protein faster than fat. Excess

What Is Alcohol?

There are many kinds of alcohol, but only one that is part of the human diet: ethanol, a colorless liquid. When yeast feed on almost any carbohydrate, they produce two waste products: ethanol and carbon dioxide. Barley and hops yield beer; grapes, wine; grains, distilled spirits such as whiskey, scotch, gin or vodka; cane sugar, rum; honey, mead; agave cactus, tequila. A standard serving of an alcoholic beverage is around ½ ounce of pure (200-proof) alcohol, 1 ounce of brandy or cognac, 1½ ounces of 80-proof distilled spirits (gin, vodka, whiskey, rum), 5 ounces of wine, or 12 ounces of regular beer.

fat calories are then efficiently converted into body fat. Wine with dinner has the same effect, the Cambridge group found, and women respond the same way as men.

The combination of alcohol, high-fat foods, and excess calories is especially fattening.

Is it the beer or the pizza that makes a beer belly? It's both, working together as a metabolic team. Yet it's only a concern if you consume more calories than you need. Says Harvard School of Public Health professor Eric Rimm, "If you are drinking beer and eating pizza, you could just as well call it a pizza belly."

DOES ALCOHOL AFFECT HOW MUCH YOU EAT?

When you have a drink, do you eat less at meals, to compensate for those extra calories? Or do you eat as much as or even more than you would normally, so alcohol's calories add to the total? Unfortunately, it's the latter:

Calories from alcoholic beverages add on to the calories from food.

In Atlanta, when moderate drinkers kept food diaries for 10 days—5 days with alcohol and 5 without—they reported taking in 200 calories more of food on days that included alcoholic beverages. On those days, their meals were larger, and lasted longer. Social occasions, with groups of friends, can encourage us both to eat more and to drink more, research shows. So keep in mind that social occasions with delicious high-fat foods and alcoholic beverages can be particularly dangerous for the weight-conscious.

THE APERITIF EFFECT

The Oxford English Dictionary defines *aperitif* as "an alcoholic drink taken before a meal as an appetizer." Dietitians frequently suggest that a drink before a meal can increase food intake in elderly men and women with poor appetites. Can a cocktail really prime the appetite?

Yes, it can. At Laval University in Ste-Foy, Quebec, Canada, men had an appetizer with wine or with juice before lunch; both appetizers had about 300 calories. On the days when the men had the appetizer with the wine, they consumed an additional 200 calories at lunch. In England, a gin-and-tonic before dinner meant people ate more. In the Netherlands, wine before lunch had a similar effect. So an aperitif does stimulate appetite. "Alcohol promotes overeating," says Laval nutrition professor Angelo Tremblay.

If you are consciously restricting calories, alcohol may cause you to lose your resolve to eat less. In the 1970s, American researchers offered women either an alcoholic beverage or a similarly flavored nonalcoholic one—and then ice cream. The women who were concerned about their body weight and who normally restrained their eating lost this restraint and ate more after they consumed the alcoholic drink. For women who didn't restrain their food intake to control weight, alcohol had no such effect. For the weight-conscious, then, alcohol can be doubly risky: *Alcoholic beverages are not only high in calories but they can break down resolve to moderate food intake.*

THE NIGHTCAP

Drinking in the evening may be the most caloric pattern of all. At Johns Hopkins University in Baltimore, a group led by Richard Foltin asked young men to live in a residential laboratory for several days, drinking the equivalent of 4 extra beverages on some days. The drinks tasted similar, but some contained alcohol while others had equivalent calories from sugar. On days in which the men drank either type of extra beverage, they consumed more total calories. One pattern of drinking was associated with increased calories in particular: *Drinks, either sugary or alcoholic, were the most likely to add extra calories to the daily total when they were consumed in the evening.*

"When people drink late in the evening, they don't compensate for the calories," says Foltin. If you drink in the evening, you'll just add those calories on to your daily total, and the next day eat as many calories as you normally do. "Drinking late in the evening is a common pattern," he says. "It may be these individuals who will wind up gaining weight."

Alcohol and Health

If you drink moderately—up to 1 daily drink for a woman, 2 for a man—chances are the habit is improving your health. The main reason is your heart. "There is overwhelming evidence that alcohol in moderation lowers the risk of coronary disease," says Harvard's Eric Rimm. Because heart disease is the most common cause of death, that translates into about a 25 percent lower risk of mortality for moderate consumers compared to abstainers. Although red wine has healthful antioxidants, it is alcohol itself that's preventing heart attacks.

For women, however, breast cancer has been a concern. "Alcohol does marginally increase the risk of breast cancer," says Rimm. Yet an average woman's risk of dying from heart disease is ten times greater than her risk of dying from breast cancer. If you are a woman at high breast cancer risk (a strong family history, for example), you may want to cut back to 1 or 2 drinks a week, he suggests. At that level, there is little or no additional risk, with some cardiovascular benefit.

If you drink *immoderately*, you can harm your health. Bingeing on 6 or more drinks even once can increase heart attack risk, and people who consistently average 3 or more drinks a day have higher rates of heart disease, stroke, certain cancers, accidents, violence, suicide, and dying prematurely. Certain people should never drink: children, adolescents, individuals who have liver disease, and, of course, alcoholics. Pregnant woman should also abstain. The dangers of drinking and driving are also very well established. Yet for the majority of Americans who drink moderately, the habit may make life both longer and healthier.

SMART STRATEGIES

We're only just beginning to understand the links between specific alcoholic beverages and food choices. We all know that certain foods "go" with particular beverages—beer with nuts or chips while watching a game on TV, cocktails with appetizers, wine with a fine dinner. "My advice is to think about how what you are drinking might affect how you are eating," says Richard Foltin. "If drinking a beer means you are going to crave potato chips, that could throw off your whole pattern. A cocktail party with high-calorie, high-fat foods is particularly risky."

How do *you* drink? What do you eat when you drink? Does a drink mean you'll lose your restraint and eat more at a party? Whether, or how, you include alcohol in your diet is a personal decision. For some individuals, alcohol is a hidden source of calories, something they don't consider when looking at their diets, and alcohol may be linked with lifestyle habits that make weight management difficult.

Several years ago, I (Bob) found myself working out next to a 28-year-old man who volunteered that he'd lost 17 pounds over 6 weeks simply by cutting out beer. Just that? As it turned out, no. He stopped going to bars with friends two or three times a week,

The Calories in a Drink

Alcohol calories can be sneaky. In particular, watch out for mixed drinks, which also contain extra calories from other ingredients, notably sugar (notice the relatively high energy density of a daiquiri or a margarita compared to beer or wine). The serving sizes for the alcoholic beverages listed below are in fluid ounces; 12 ounces is a cup and a half, or ¾ pint; some brands may differ slightly in calories. While we provide the energy density of each beverage, use it to compare beverages, not, for instance, to compare a beer and an apple; we regulate beverage intake differently from food intake. Watch portions, too: A pint-size pina colada in a bar or restaurant is actually 4 "servings," with more than 1,000 calories!

Beverage	Serving Size	Weight (grams)	Calories	Energy Density
Beer	12 ounces	356	160	0.4
Light beer	12 ounces	354	100	0.3
Nonalcoholic beer	12 ounces	360	32	0.1
Red wine	4 ounces	118	85	0.7
White wine	4 ounces	118	80	0.7
Wine cooler	8 ounces	240	120	0.5
Daiquiri	4 ounces	121	225	1.9
Margarita	4 ounces	124	270	2.2
Gin-and-tonic	4 ounces	120	150	0.7
Pina colada	4 ounces	141	262	1.9

drinking 5 or 6 beers each night, eating pizza, and often feeling too tired to work out the next morning. He started to eat fewer snacks and more nutritious foods, started walking 1–2 hours 5 days a week, and lifting weights three times a week. When I talked with him, he was going out for beers only about once every 2 weeks or so, and had cut back to 2 beers on each occasion.

If you want to include alcohol in a calorie-controlled plan, you'll need to incorporate such beverages into a consumption pattern that minimizes their tendency to add extra calories. One such pattern may be to drink moderately with meals, rather than between meals with caloric snacks. At Colorado State University in Fort Collins, young men were asked to include 2 glasses of wine and no other alcohol with their evening meal for 6 weeks. For the next 6 weeks, they abstained from alcohol. They ate whatever and wherever they usually did. In this naturalistic study, drinking moderately with meals did *not* increase total calories. Such a pattern may also be the healthiest.

"The rule I go by is, I only drink with meals," says Foltin. "It keeps me from drinking too much. And it may also keep me from eating too much." He believes that people are better able to compensate for alcohol's calories by eating less when they consume beverages with a meal. Says Tremblay, "How alcohol affects weight depends on the rest of the diet. If you have a glass of wine or beer with your dinner of soup, lean steak, green vegetables, and fruit salad for dessert, there will be no overeating. The wine or beer is paired with other ingredients that promote satiety with fewer calories."

SUMMARY

- With 7 calories per gram, alcohol is high in energy density, making it easy to consume excess calories.

- Combining alcoholic beverages with high-fat, energy-dense foods promotes weight gain.

- Alcohol's calories add on to the calories from food. When we drink, we often eat about as much food at meals as when we don't drink.

- Alcohol lowers inhibitions, including those against overeating. This poses a particular problem for people who normally restrain their eating to control weight.

- Drinking late in the evening is a pattern that may promote extra daily calories.

- Pay attention to the foods you eat when you drink. If drinking a beer makes you reach for the chips, you'll need either to change that association, or to drink beer less frequently.

- If you drink, the best pattern for weight and health is to consume wine or beer with a filling meal that's low in energy density.

Water and Other Beverages

Water taken in moderation cannot hurt anybody.
—MARK TWAIN, *Notebook*

WATER PLAYS A CRITICAL ROLE in *Volumetrics*. It has weight but no calories: Its energy density is zero. To lower the energy density of your diet, you'll want to eat more naturally water-rich foods, such as fruits and vegetables, as well as dishes that incorporate water, such as hot cereals, pasta, rice, steamed or poached fish, casseroles, soups, stews, and low-fat frozen desserts.

But what about beverages? Can you go further and simply consume a large portion of your diet in liquid form? Wouldn't drinks be even more effective than solid foods in helping you feel full?

It's not that simple.

Are You Getting Enough Water?

Humans aren't like camels. We can't store water. We need to replenish fluids daily. How much do we need? The National Research Council recommends about a quart (4 cups) for every 1,000 calories expended. That's about 12 cups for a man, 9 for a woman. You need more if you spend much time outside in the heat or are very active. Fiber also increases water needs.

It needn't all come from drinking plain water. We also get water from fruit juice, milk, carbonated beverages, and foods. A typical balanced diet of 2,000 calories contains 2–3 cups of water in the food. You'll also get water in beverages that are caffeinated (coffee, tea, colas) or alcoholic (beer, wine), although you lose some, because alcohol and caffeine act as diuretics, increasing the body's loss of water as urine.

For most people, thirst is the best way to know that you need to drink more fluids. But there are exceptions:

- **Intense exercise, especially in hot weather.** You may lose fluids so quickly that by the time your thirst mechanism kicks in, you may already be a little dehydrated. Drink 2 cups of water in the 2 hours before exercise, and drink between ½ cup and 1 cup every 15 minutes or so while you exercise.

- **Age.** The elderly have a blunted sense of thirst. In the Eating Lab, when young and elderly men consumed no fluids overnight, the next day the young men were very thirsty and rapidly drank enough water to restore fluid balance. But the elderly men experienced little thirst and drank so little water they remained dehydrated. Older readers should take care that they drink enough fluids when they are ill, exercising, or overheated.

One indicator of the adequacy of fluid intake is the color of the urine: It should be pale yellow. If your urine is often very concentrated and dark yellow in color, try to drink more water.

Water and many beverages quench thirst but don't satisfy hunger. Simply drinking water with a meal won't help you eat less at the meal, or at the next one, we've found in controlled studies. But water *will* quench your thirst without calories, and that can help you satisfy your need for liquid without adding calories to your diet.

WATER WON'T FILL YOU UP

Have you ever heard that drinking water is a good way to stave off hunger? It's a common belief. "To stave off the rigors of feeling famished," wrote food writer M. F. K. Fisher in *A Cordiall Water* in the 1960s, "drink something very thin and watery, like cold weak coffee from a bottle, or wine cut with at least five times its amount of water, or water with a little vinegar in it."

We're not sure where this idea originated, but it has been tested, and found wanting. Controlled experiments have concluded that drinking water before a meal or drinking extra water with a meal has no effect on food intake. Water may simply empty from the stomach too quickly to affect satiety. The bottom line: *People eat the same amount at lunch or dinner whether they drink extra water or not.*

CAN YOU MISTAKE THIRST FOR HUNGER?

You see it all the time in tips for dieters: "You may be eating because you are thirsty, not hungry." We're skeptical.

The body senses hunger and thirst through separate mechanisms. Hunger mechanisms detect changes in the level of body fuels such as blood sugar (glucose). On the other hand, thirst mechanisms respond to signals such as increases in blood levels of sodium or decreases in blood volume. When you drink water or other beverages, these dilute the sodium and increase blood volume and you feel less thirsty. If you eat food, especially if it's salty or sugary, you'll feel *more* thirsty. Because hunger and thirst are controlled by different mechanisms, it is unlikely that you are eating more food because you are thirsty.

One reason people may confuse thirst and hunger is that they often occur at the same time, around meal times. Nearly three quarters of beverage consumption occurs with food. To satisfy both needs, you should drink beverages that contain few or no calories, and low-energy-dense foods for hunger. Another reason people may mistake thirst for hunger is that they have an urge for something in their mouths. If this happens to you, you should find strategies that help you control thirst, such as chewing gum, which increases salivation, or sipping water or other low-calorie drinks.

The Health Benefits of Water

Water helps every cell in the body. It helps move food through the digestive tract, carry nutrients from the gut into the blood and to the cells, and eliminate waste products. It's critical for maintaining body temperature. It lubricates joints and gives form to cells. Yet many of us take in too little.

"At least half of Americans are mildly dehydrated," says Susan M. Kleiner of the University of Washington, Seattle. Symptoms include mild fatigue, slight headache, dry throat, or dry cough. It's well established that drinking enough water helps prevent kidney stones (even in people who have already passed one). There may be a cancer protective link, too. Men who drink more than 6 glasses of water a day are 50 percent less likely to develop bladder cancer than men who drink less than 1 glass a day, find Harvard researchers. Adequate fluid intake may also help to lower the risk of colon and breast cancer.

By following *Volumetrics*, you'll already consume more water-rich foods like fruits, vegetables, and soup. Drinking more water is another positive health action.

THE SODA TRAP

For weight management, the biggest benefit to drinking water is that it will help you escape a common caloric trap: drinking high-calorie beverages when you are actually thirsty, not hungry. Soft drinks will satisfy thirst, although not as well as water. Anything liquid, especially if it is cool, decreases thirst. But with soft drinks you'll be consuming extra calories that will do little to provide satiety, so you'll eat just as much.

Our bodies respond to sugary soft drinks primarily as thirst-quenching liquids, so we don't regulate their calories efficiently. This has been demonstrated over and over again: Sugar-laden drinks have little effect on how much people eat at a meal, or over several meals, or even over several weeks. They add calories to your daily total. When we gave men a pint of lemonade with 166 calories either an hour before, 30 minutes before, or during lunch, it had no impact on how many calories from food they consumed at lunch–the drink calories were added to the total. It doesn't matter whether drinks are carbonated or noncarbonated, or whether the sugar is sucrose or high-fructose corn syrup. They all add extra calories. Dietary surveys at Georgia State University found that meal by meal, day by day, people ate as much food whether they drank caloric beverages or not.

Soft drink consumption has been rising for decades, with no end in sight. In the 1950s, Coca-Cola was sold only in a 6½-ounce bottle. Now a standard-size bottle is 20 ounces. These supersizes make it easy to gulp down huge quantities. A 32-ounce soda from a fast-food restaurant can easily top 500 calories. The Center for Science in the Public Interest, a public interest group, calculates that on average, every adult American drinks more than one and a half 12-ounce cans of soda every day. That's more than twice the amount as in 1974. Only about a quarter are diet soft drinks. Nutrition surveys reveal that adults who are heavy consumers of soft drinks take in more calories than adults who drink fewer such beverages.

Those extra calories can lead to weight gain. When men and women were asked by researchers at the Monell Chemical Senses Center in Philadelphia to drink about 3½ sodas a day for 3 weeks, the men gained 2 pounds; the women, 1. When they drank diet sodas, the women stayed the same weight, while the men lost a pound. The bottom line: *Don't drink sugary soft drinks to quench your thirst. They'll add calories to your daily total.*

SMART CHOICES

To quench thirst, drink water. A low-calorie or calorie-free drink, as long as it is also caffeine- and alcohol-free, is another good choice. Skip sports drinks, which are highly caloric. If you want caffeine, coffee or tea is okay, but watch the calories from the added milk and sugar; some large cold sweetened coffee drinks can top 500 calories. If you really want the taste of a caloric drink such as a soft drink, and can afford the calories, enjoy one in a small portion. Think of it as a snack or dessert.

What about fruit juice? Even 100 percent pure fruit juices contain plenty of sugar and thus calories. Some juices like orange or grapefruit are nutritious, though, so you should continue to drink

Instead of Soda . . .

A standard 12-ounce soft drink averages 150 calories. Those calories can add up. What can you drink instead? One alternative is a diet soda. Here are more:

- **Water.** Substituting water for caloric drinks is an easy way to cut calories. In our studies, it's also a better thirst quencher than sugary drinks. Mineral water or seltzer is also calorie-free, but watch out for "flavored" seltzers, which can contain as many calories as soft drinks.

- **Iced tea.** Skip the canned stuff; it's loaded with sugar and calories. Make your own iced tea by putting two tea bags, along with 1½ tablespoons sugar (and a sprig of mint if you have it) in 1½ cups cold water in a tall glass on a sunny window. Cover it and let it sit for 20 minutes. Remove tea bags, add ice, and enjoy. Calories: 60. Try iced herbal teas, too.

- **Lemonade.** Instead of caloric canned or bottled versions, squeeze the juice of 1 lemon into a canning jar with a lid. In a microwave-safe cup, bring ¼ cup water with 1½ tablespoons sugar in it to a boil in the microwave. Now add the sugar syrup to the lemon juice in the jar along with a cup of cold tap water, plus the lemon rinds. Put the cover back on and shake; serve in a tall glass over ice. Calories: 60.

- **Fruit juice spritzers.** Add seltzer to orange juice, grapefruit juice, or other fruit juices. With 1 cup seltzer and ½ cup orange juice, you'll have 60 calories. With grapefruit juice, it's 50; with pineapple, 70. You may even want to experiment with adding seltzer to soft drinks like ginger ale to cut calories.

- **Hot, hot, hot.** Hot tea with lemon, low-fat hot chocolate sweetened with a sugar substitute, hot lemonade, and other such beverages can be sipped slowly, providing a sensory experience that lasts a long time.

---

them; aim for ¾ cup (6 ounces), a volume you may want to boost with zero-calorie club soda. Juices with pulp may be more satiating than clear juices, but we don't have firm evidence. We do know that whole fruit is more satiating than fruit juices. Apples, oranges, and grapes are more satiating than apple juice, orange juice, or grape juice respectively. So don't skip juice, but make sure you also eat whole fruit.

Some beverages *can* satisfy hunger. They cross over the line from being a drink that just quenches thirst to being a food that satisfies hunger. Vegetable juice, like V–8, is one example. When we gave young men nearly a pint (14 ounces, 88 calories) of vegetable juice before lunch, they took in 136 fewer calories at the meal. "Tomato juice is actually a suspension, not a liquid like soda," explains medicine professor Kenneth Koch of Penn State College of Medicine. "There is some residual in the stomach, and that slows stomach emptying." That, in turn, increases satiety.

Milk-based drinks are also satiating. They help people feel full and eat less at the next meal, we've found. "Milk turns to a semisolid in the stomach," explains Koch. "There's more neuromuscular work that must be done, which increases the satiety signals going to the brain that say that you're not on empty any more. When you

The Water in Food

Not all water is found in a glass. Many "solid" foods are largely water, too. Such foods play a big role in *Volumetrics*: When water is incorporated into a food, it is more satiating than when water is consumed as a beverage. Many of the low-energy-dense foods you'll be eating are good sources of water.

Food	Water Content
Fruits and vegetables	80–95 percent
Hot cereal	85 percent
Egg, boiled	75 percent
Pasta	65 percent
Fish and seafood	60–85 percent
Meats	45–65 percent
Bread	35–40 percent
Cheese	35 percent
Nuts	2–5 percent
Oil	0 percent

Source: *Bowes & Church's Food Values of Portions Commonly Used*, 17th edition (Lippincott, 1998).

How to Lower Energy Density Using Water-Rich Foods

- Eat fruit with breakfast: half a grapefruit, an orange, an apple, or a banana. Make a fruit salad with two or more of your favorite fruits.

- Top cereals, pancakes, and waffles with fruits such as peaches, blueberries, strawberries, or raspberries.

- For a snack, choose fresh fruit rather than dried fruit, or baked or fried food.

- Add vegetables such as zucchini, yellow squash, peppers, onions, eggplant, and spinach to pasta dishes and pizza.

- Add extra vegetables to sandwiches.

- Increase the proportion of vegetables in stir-fry dishes, fajitas, soups, and stews.

- Start lunch or dinner with a bowl of broth-based soup.

- Include a tossed green salad or fruit salad with dinner.

- Choose desserts that contain fruit.

---

drink a glass of milk, you're not hungry for a while." That's true for skim milk as well as whole milk, and for frothy skim milk–based drinks like low-fat milkshakes.

Surprisingly, the more dilute the milk drinks, the greater the suppression of later food intake, we've found in our studies. This effect is related to the volume of the drinks. When calories are held constant, increasing the volume and reducing the energy density of the drinks by the addition of water increases the effect of the drinks on satiety. The same phenomenon holds true with soup, as you'll see in the next chapter.

SUMMARY

- Water satisfies thirst, not hunger. You won't eat less if you drink water before or during a meal. To increase satiety, incorporate low-energy-dense, water-rich foods into your diet.

- When you're thirsty, limit consumption of highly caloric beverages such as soft drinks. They add calories to your diet without satisfying hunger, which can lead to weight gain.

- To quench thirst, water is the best choice, followed by low-calorie or calorie-free beverages such as seltzer-diluted fruit juice, a diet soft drink, or herbal tea.

- Thicker drinks, such as a vegetable cocktail, and drinks containing protein, such as those based on milk, satisfy hunger. These "liquid foods" are good choices for increased satiety.

Soup

I live on good soup, not fine words.
— MOLIÈRE

SOUP IS A FOOD YOU DRINK. It's mostly water. Yet our bodies perceive it as food, not drink. Soup based on broth, rather than cream or a starchy puree, is at the low end of the energy-density spectrum.

The satiety difference between water consumed on its own as a beverage and as an ingredient in soup is remarkable. We demonstrated this when we gave women a 270-calorie first course before lunch. On some days, the women got a chicken-rice casserole. On others, they got the same casserole plus a 10-ounce glass of water. On another occasion, they got the casserole with an extra 10 ounces of water cooked into it to make soup. It was only the soup that reduced the calories they ate at the lunch that followed (see p. 100).

Not only did the women consume about 100 calories less at lunch after the soup, they didn't feel hungrier later, and didn't eat more at dinner to make up the difference. In Paris, experimenters recently reported the same thing: Water as a beverage with a meal

The Soup Experiments

Drinking water with a casserole doesn't reduce calories consumed—but adding water to casserole to make soup does.

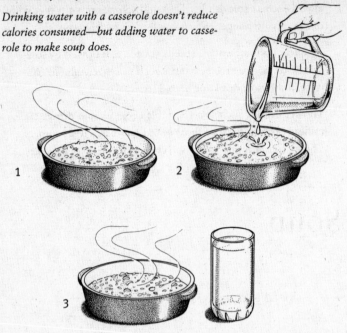

1 *Chicken-rice-vegetable casserole. E.D.: 0.8. Serving size: 1⅓ cup. Calories consumed at lunch: 392.*

2 *Chicken-rice-vegetable soup. E.D.: 0.4. Serving size: 2½ cups. Calories consumed at lunch: 289.*

3 *Chicken-rice-vegetable casserole. E.D.: 0.8. Plus 10-ounce glass of water. Serving size: 1⅓ cup food, 2½ cups including water. Calories consumed at lunch: 396.*

didn't enhance satiety, but the same ingredients made into soup did. Chunky soup, they found, was more satiating than strained soup.

"The stomach empties liquids differently from solids, and lighter, more dilute liquids differently from heavier ones," says Penn State professor Kenneth Koch. "The water you drink is long gone by the time a water-containing food like soup empties from the stomach." Soup may contain some fat that slows its release from the stomach, and it also contains pieces of solid food, either tiny or in big chunks, that the stomach needs to break down further before sending it on to the intestines. "When you cook a noodle, it absorbs water, but your stomach no longer recognizes that as water—it now identifies it as a noodle," he says.

So the next time you feel hungry, try a large soothing bowl of broth-based soup. If you have it as a first course before lunch, it will be easier to eat fewer calories for your lunch, and you probably won't eat more at dinner. If you have it as a first course before dinner, you'll likely eat less at that meal, too.

TO DROP WEIGHT, PICK UP YOUR SOUP SPOON

In the early 1980s, Henry Jordan, M.D., then at the University of Pennsylvania, asked 500 people in a weight loss program to record every meal they ate for 10 weeks. Some were instructed to eat soup at least four times a week. The more soup they ate, the fewer calories they took in and the more weight they lost. On average, they consumed 100 fewer calories a day compared to people who had soup less frequently.

Eating more soup also helps you keep weight off. At Baylor College of Medicine in Houston, overweight men and women on a low-calorie diet who were instructed to eat soup every day liked the strategy better than those just reducing calories, and they maintained their weight loss better over the following year. "Soup works," says Baylor's John Foreyt. "It helps people to eat less."

SOUP AND SATIETY

"Beautiful soup, so rich and green, waiting in a hot tureen!" wrote Lewis Carroll in *Alice's Adventures in Wonderland* (1865). "Who for such dainties would not stoop?" If it's a good soup, hearty but not heavy, it will fill you up, give pleasure to your tongue and mouth and nose, deliver a visual message to your brain that a large satisfying food is about to be eaten, and activate a series of biological signals that tell you that you've had enough to eat.

The main reason is soup's low energy density. At the Eating Lab, we found that when we gave people a broth-based soup before lunch, they ate less than if we gave the same number of calories in an appetizer of cheese and crackers. It's not surprising, once you realize that a 200-calorie pre-lunch snack of cheese and crackers weighs only 1½ ounces while our soup weighed 20 ounces (2½ cups). We know it is not soup's temperature that is responsible for its satiating power—cold soup worked just as well as hot soup.

Soup evokes satiety in just about every way we know a food can. When you start a meal with a cup or more of soup, you see a reasonable portion in front of you. This visual cue leads you to expect that it will be filling. The same phenomenon happens when we eat a big portion of any food of low energy density, whether it's a salad or a bowl of cereal with fruit.

Now you have your first sip. If you like it, you'll experience pleasurable sensory stimulation: the aromas that waft into your nose, the tastes of sweet and sour and bitter and salty on your tongue, the warmth as you swallow. With a big portion of low-density soup, you get a lot of sensory stimulation. We know from our studies that the more sensory stimulation you get from a food, the more satisfying it is. We need a certain amount of chewing, savoring, smelling, tasting, and swallowing to feel that we've eaten enough of a particular food.

As you swallow spoonful after spoonful of the delicious soup, it moves down your throat into your stomach, where its big volume fills up your stomach. It activates the stomach's "stretch receptors," sending satiety messages to the brain. The more food, the more of these messages get conveyed. "Even if the calories are low, if you consume a big weight of food, your stomach still has to do the same amount of work, and it takes the same amount of time," says Koch.

As the soup empties from your stomach, satiety hormones are released into the blood, which help us feel full. If you eat soup with high-fiber whole grains and vegetables, as well as meat, it will leave the stomach slowly. As the soup is digested, some of its calories are converted into blood sugar (glucose), which causes insulin levels to rise, and these also provide the body with signals about how much food has been eaten. This exquisite sequence of events, which follows eating, is critical for satiety.

Soup is an ideal food for activating these mechanisms. Is it unique? Of course not. Any food that's low in energy density will allow you to consume a satisfying portion and reduce hunger with relatively few calories. If you don't like soup, start your meal with a salad, a piece of fruit, a glass of vegetable juice, or any first course that's low in energy density.

SOUP STRATEGIES

Don't even think of living on just soup. When I (Barbara) appeared on the ABC program *20/20* in 1998, explaining the principles that would form the basis of this book, the segment began with a profile of a woman on the "cabbage soup" diet. Whenever she was hungry, she explained, she was supposed to eat cabbage soup, morning, noon, or night. She looked miserable! Several months later, when she was reinterviewed, she had regained the weight lost on that diet. If you follow such a highly restrictive diet, you may eat less for a while out of sheer boredom, but you will not be able to sustain such a strategy.

If you like soup, on the other hand, you may find it enjoyable to eat it frequently. Have it as a first course, or as a main meal. Open a can, pop a paper container in a microwave, order it when you're eating out, or make your own, perhaps freezing it in single servings you can microwave when you want a bowl. Soup is only part of the answer to eating fewer calories while enjoying one of life's pleasures: food. Soup-only diets don't work. But soup does.

SUMMARY

- Eating soup as a first course will help you to eat less and lose weight.

- Broth-based soup is very low in energy density so you can eat a satisfying portion with few calories.

- Water, which lowers the energy density of a food, must be incorporated into the food to enhance satiety.

- Eat broth-based soup, as a first course or as the basis for a meal, as often as you feel is practical for you, or start your meals with other low-energy-dense foods, like salad, vegetable juice, or a piece of fruit.

200 Calories of Soup

If you're watching calories, soup is *almost* always a good choice. It depends on the kind: If it's broth-based, it will be low in energy density, but if it's cream-based, all bets are off. For each soup below, we'll list the energy density and show you how much you can eat for 200 calories:

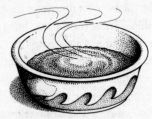

Cream of broccoli with cheese.
E.D.: 0.8. Serving size: 1 cup.
This cream-based soup with lots of cheese is the highest in energy density, so the portion is small.

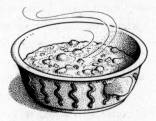

New England clam chowder.
E.D.: 0.7. Serving size: 1¼ cup.
This classic cream soup also provides a small portion.

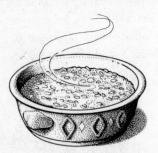

Chicken-rice.
E.D.: 0.5. Serving size: 1¾ cup.
A good choice: it's very low in energy density and provides a filling portion.

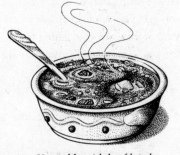

Vegetable with beef broth.
E.D.: 0.3. Serving size: 2½ cups.
With plenty of water-rich vegetables, this one is even lower in energy density, so the portion is larger.

WHAT ARE THE BEST FOOD CHOICES for weight management? By now you know the importance of choosing foods that are lower in energy density so you can maintain satisfying portions. In this section, we'll show you the energy densities of a wide spectrum of common foods, so you can make smart choices.

The energy densities of foods fall into four broad categories:

Category 1: Very Low-Energy-Dense Foods. These are foods that supply less than 0.6 calories per gram. In general, you can consume large amounts of foods from this category without consuming too many calories. This category includes most fruits and vegetables, skim milk, and broth-based soups. The more foods you eat from this category, the greater likelihood that you will lower the overall energy density of your dietary pattern. In particular, you can eat large portions of whole fruits, and vegetables with no added fat. (The big exception in this category: caloric beverages, which are often very low in energy density—both regular beer and cola drinks average 0.4 calories per gram—but can supply calories without satisfying hunger, and so should be limited in a weight management program.)

Category 2: Low-Energy-Dense Foods. These are foods that supply from 0.6 to 1.5 calories per gram. This is a very important category; most of your food choices should come from this group, which includes many cooked grains, many breakfast cereals (when served with low-fat 1 percent or fat-free milk), low-fat meats, legumes (dry beans, peas, chickpeas, lima beans, soybeans, lentils), many mixed dishes, salads, cottage cheese, and fat-free salad dressings. While you can't eat as much as you want from this category if you're watching calories, you can consume relatively large portions of foods.

Category 3: Medium-Energy-Dense Foods. These are foods that supply from 1.5 to 4.0 calories per gram. This is a broad category that includes a wide variety of foods: meats, cheeses, some mixed dishes, salad dressings, some snack foods, and some desserts. Choose more foods from the lower end of this category. You'll want to be very careful of portion size of foods at the higher end of this category, because they can be easily overeaten.

Category 4: High-Energy-Dense Foods. These are foods that supply from 4.0 calories per gram to 9.0 calories per gram, which is as energy dense as a food can get. This category includes crackers, chips, chocolate candies, frostings, cookies, nuts, butter, and full-fat condiments. You'll need to manage your consumption of foods from this category very carefully. You can do so by substituting foods from a lower-energy-density category (e.g., low-fat mayo for full-fat mayo) or by consciously limiting portion size (2 teaspoons rather than 2 tablespoons of peanut butter). Some of these foods, such as nuts, are nutritious, so consuming small portions is a healthful strategy.

The Energy Density Spectrum below should provide you with a good general idea of how common foods fall into these four categories. (We'll give you more complete information in the charts that follow on pp. 116–148.) But energy density shouldn't be your only guide to choosing foods. The best nutritional guidance for choosing a healthful diet remains the United States Department of Agriculture's Food Guide Pyramid. Next, we'll show you how to follow the Pyramid the *Volumetric* way.

THE ENERGY DENSITY SPECTRUM FOR SELECTED FOODS

Category 1: Very Low-Energy-Dense Foods (0 to 0.6 calories per gram)

Water	0.0
Lettuce	0.1
Tomato	0.2
Strawberry	0.2
Broccoli (cooked)	0.3
Salsa	0.3
Grapefruit	0.3
Vegetarian vegetable soup	0.3
Cantaloupe	0.4
Milk, skim	0.4
Winter squash	0.4
Applesauce	0.4
Carrots	0.4
Chicken, rice, and vegetable soup	0.5

Italian dressing, fat-free	0.5
Orange	0.5
Yogurt, fat-free with aspartame	0.5
Vegetarian chili	0.5
Yogurt, fat-free, plain	0.6
Blueberries	0.6
Apples	0.6

Category 2: Low-Energy-Dense Foods (0.6 to 1.5 calories per gram)

Tofu	0.6
Milk, whole	0.6
Oatmeal, prepared with water	0.6
Mayonnaise, fat-free	0.6
Cottage cheese, fat-free	0.7
Grapes	0.7
Black beans	0.8
Green peas	0.8
Corn on the cob (boiled, drained)	0.9
Orange roughy (broiled)	0.9
Banana	0.9
Sour cream, fat-free	0.9
Yogurt, 99 percent fat-free	1.0
Pudding, vanilla, prepared with 2 percent milk	1.0
Cottage cheese, regular (full-fat)	1.0
Cheerios with 1 percent milk	1.1
Tuna, canned in water	1.1
Crispix with 1 percent milk	1.1
Potato, baked with skin	1.1
Veal chop, braised	1.2
Yogurt, fat-free, vanilla	1.2
Frozen yogurt, fruit varieties	1.3
Rice, white, long-grain, cooked	1.3
Ham, extra lean, 5 percent fat	1.3
Turkey breast, roasted, no skin	1.4
Ranch dressing, fat-free	1.4
Spaghetti, cooked	1.5

Category 3: Medium-Energy-Dense Foods (1.5 to 4.0 calories per gram)

Egg, hard boiled	1.6
Chicken breast, roasted, no skin	1.7
Hummus	1.7
Ham, 11 percent fat	1.8
Sirloin steak, lean, broiled	1.9
Pork chop, center loin, broiled	2.0
Pumpkin pie	2.1
Margarine, low-calorie	2.1
Apricots, dried	2.4
Bread, whole-wheat	2.5
Grape jelly	2.5
English muffin	2.6
Angel food cake	2.6
Mozzarella cheese, part-skim	2.6
Ranch dressing, reduced-fat	2.7
Potato chips, fat-free	2.7
Italian bread, white	2.7
Bagel, plain	2.8
Raisins	3.0
Potatoes, French-fried	3.2
Mayonnaise, light	3.3
Donut, jelly-filled	3.4
Cream cheese, full-fat	3.5
Fruit chewy cookies	3.6
Italian dressing, full-fat	3.6
Butter, light	3.6
Chocolate cake with frosting	3.7
Licorice, cherry	3.7
Swiss cheese	3.8
Hard pretzels	3.8
Popcorn, air-popped, plain	3.8
Rice cakes, plain	3.9
Tortilla chips, baked	3.9

Graham crackers	4.2
Chocolate chip cookies, homemade	4.6
Tortilla chips	4.6
Creme-filled chocolate sandwich cookies	4.9
M&M's, plain	4.9
Bacon	5.0
Potato chips	5.4
Milk chocolate bar	5.4
Peanuts, roasted	5.9
Ranch dressing, full-fat	5.9
Peanut butter, creamy	5.9
Pecans, dry roasted	6.6
Mayonnaise, regular, full-fat	7.1
Butter	7.2
Margarine, stick	7.2
Oil, vegetable	8.8

Volumetrics and the Food Guide Pyramid

VOLUMETRICS ENHANCES SOUND NUTRITION. It is consistent with the United States Department of Agriculture's Food Guide Pyramid *(opposite)*.

The Food Guide Pyramid is particularly good at demonstrating the best *proportion* of the food groups in a balanced diet. The "base" of our diet should be breads, cereals, rice, and pasta. The next tier is composed of vegetable and fruits, which we should eat in abundance. But we need smaller portions from the next tier, which is composed of dairy foods (milk, yogurt, cheese) and pro-

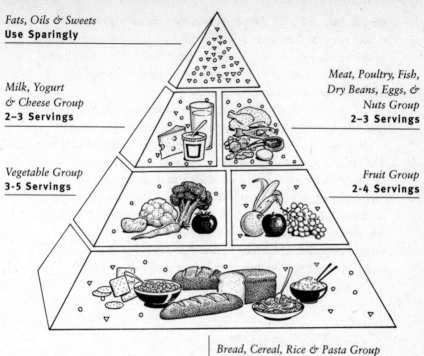

Fats, Oils & Sweets
Use Sparingly

Milk, Yogurt
& Cheese Group
2–3 Servings

Vegetable Group
3-5 Servings

Meat, Poultry, Fish,
Dry Beans, Eggs, &
Nuts Group
2–3 Servings

Fruit Group
2-4 Servings

Bread, Cereal, Rice & Pasta Group
6-11 Servings

tein-rich foods (meat; poultry; fish; legumes, including dry beans; eggs; and nuts. The smallest tier is fats, oils, and sweets, foods we should eat sparingly. The Pyramid recommends that we consume 6–11 daily servings from the breads, cereals, rice, and pasta group; 3–5 from the vegetables group; 2–4 from the fruits group; 2–3 from the milk, yogurt, and cheese group; and 2–3 from the meat, poultry, fish, legumes, eggs, and nuts group. The range is based on calorie needs. If you are consuming 1,600 calories a day, you'll take in the smaller number from that range, for example.

For weight management, however, the Pyramid isn't a complete guide. It leaves out a crucial piece of information: energy density. This is not a criticism of the Pyramid, which wasn't designed to guide you toward lower-calorie choices, but as a graphic illustration of a healthful, balanced diet. It still serves this purpose, which is why we include it. But for weight management, energy density makes a crucial difference. It is important whether you select whole or skim milk, extra lean ham or baby back ribs, whole-wheat bread or donuts. Your choice of food within each food group will greatly affect how many calories you consume.

Serving size is also a source of great confusion with the Pyramid. Because serving size is so important to *Volumetrics,* we want to clear this up so you can use the Pyramid in making food choices. The main thing to remember is that Pyramid serving sizes are smaller than the amount of food most people eat in a portion. (The "serving size" on nutritional labels is based on typically consumed portions, and is usually bigger than Pyramid serving sizes.) A Pyramid serving is as small as a half-cup of cooked rice, pasta, or mashed potatoes; a "medium" piece of fruit the size of a tennis ball; and a piece of meat, poultry, or fish the size of a deck of cards.

Here are the sizes of those foods on your plate:

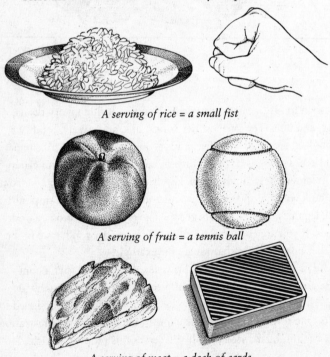

A serving of rice = a small fist

A serving of fruit = a tennis ball

A serving of meat = a deck of cards

Because serving size is smaller than most people realize, it's easy to underestimate how many servings you've eaten. So it's important to get a better understanding of serving sizes. That doesn't mean you need to limit yourself to 1 serving from a food group at a time, however. This is important, especially for foods of low energy density like fruits and vegetables. We want you to eat more of these foods; they are healthful and very low in energy density. If you eat 1½ cups of steamed broccoli with a tablespoon of low-fat lemon vinaigrette, that's 3 servings. But that's fine. It's so low in energy density that eating more than 1 serving still provides a small amount of calories, and fills you up.

Nor do you need to limit yourself to 1 serving of grain products, low-fat dairy foods, or lean protein-rich foods at any one meal. It's okay to eat a cup of rice (2 servings) rather than ½ cup (1 serving), or a 6-ounce piece of fish (2 servings) rather than 2 or 3 ounces (1 serving). But you do need to know what a serving size is, so you can figure out if your dietary pattern is balanced. Most of the confusion about Pyramid serving sizes comes from these two food groups, grains and meat, so pay particular attention. (The dairy group is easier, because most people know what a cup of milk or yogurt is.)

Most Americans consume enough foods from the grains group, too few fruits and vegetables, more than enough foods from the protein/meat group, and a little less dairy than is optimal. We also eat too much from the top of the Pyramid, the "fats, oils, and sweets" at the apex. So keep that in mind in selecting foods. If you follow *Volumetrics*, you'll be eating more fruits and vegetables, and adequate amounts from the other food groups. You'll also choose foods *within* each food group that are lower in energy density. For weight management, this is critical. In the next chapter (p. 116), we'll show you how.

What Is a Serving?

Here is how the USDA defines a serving for the five food groups in the Food Guide Pyramid.

Bread, Cereals, Rice, and Pasta Group

1 slice of bread
½ cup cooked pasta, rice, grits
½ cup hot cereal
1 ounce ready-to-eat cereal
½ English muffin
½ hamburger bun
¼ large (4- to 5-ounce) bagel
1 small roll, biscuit, or muffin
1 small (4-inch) pita
5 or 6 small crackers
3 medium breadsticks
12 tortilla chips
1 7-inch flour or corn tortilla
2 cups popcorn
⅕ of a 10-inch angel food cake

Vegetable Group

½ cup cooked vegetable
1 cup raw leafy vegetables, such as salad greens
1 medium tomato
½ cup tomato sauce
1 medium carrot
1 medium ear of corn
2 spears of broccoli
¾ cup 100 percent vegetable juice
1 cup vegetable soup

Fruit Group

¼ cup dried fruit
¼ medium cantaloupe
½ medium mango

½ medium grapefruit

½ cup canned or cooked fruit

½ cup fresh cut-up fruit

½ cup frozen fruit

½ cup strawberries or blueberries

¼ cup 100 percent fruit juice

1 large kiwi

1 medium apple

1 medium banana

1 medium orange

1 medium peach

2 medium apricots

2½ canned pineapple slices, drained

Milk, Yogurt, and Cheese Group

1 cup (8 ounces) milk

1 cup yogurt

1½ ounces natural cheese

2 ounces processed cheese

½ cup evaporated milk

1 cup frozen yogurt or low-fat ice cream, or 1½ cups ice milk

Meat, Poultry, Fish, Legumes, Eggs, and Nuts Group

2–3 ounces cooked lean beef, pork, veal, or lamb

2–3 ounces poultry without skin

2–3 ounces fish (without bones)

2–3 ounces canned fish, drained

2–3 ounces seafood

1 cup dry beans, cooked

1 cup baked beans

1 cup tofu (9 ounces)

2 eggs

4 tablespoons peanut butter

¼ cup seeds (sunflower, pumpkin)

⅓ cup nuts (almonds, walnuts, peanuts)

The Energy Density Spectrum

The main criteria to making more *Volumetric* choices within each Pyramid Food Group is energy density, abbreviated in the charts that follow as E.D. and expressed as calories per gram of food. Use this E.D. number to compare foods within each group. The charts list foods from the lowest E.D. to the highest within each food group, so it's easy to scan down and compare foods. In general, choose foods with lower E.D.'s within each food group. Thus, in the "Bread and Grain Products" chart below, Melba toast has an E.D. of 3.9, while fat-free whole-wheat tortilla has an E.D. of 1.6; that means that gram for gram and ounce for ounce, tortillas have half the calories compared to Melba toast. So fat-free whole-wheat tortillas are a better choice for satiety.

There are exceptions, of course. We measure E.D. by calories in a given weight (grams) of food, not actual volume. Some foods, like popcorn, that have a fairly high E.D. but lots of volume are actually pretty satiating foods for the calories. So you'll also want to look at the standard portion sizes we give, and the calories, to get a more complete idea of how much of a given food you can eat for the calories. Look for foods that give big portions with few calories.

Comparison is the main purpose of these charts. In most cases, we use the Food Guide Pyramid serving sizes, but in a few, we follow customary portions so you can compare between similar foods. We give breakfast cereals for a 1 cup portion, rather than 1 ounce, for instance, so you can compare the calories in the same portion. In the "Milk, Yogurt, and Cheese" chart, we give yogurt information for 6 ounces (3/4 cup), instead of 1 cup, because that's the amount of yogurt you'll typically get in a container. We list foods this way so you can compare caloric counts and energy density for similar foods.

Finally, not *every* food choice you make should be determined by energy density. Some foods of higher energy density, like nuts, are very nutritious, and you may want to include them in your diet. Others, like chocolate, are too delicious to give up. But the charts below will help you make smarter choices, so you know which foods you can eat in satisfying portions without too many calories, and which ones require careful portion management.

As a quick visual guide, we've also included energy density spectrums for each chart. The purpose of these is to let you see at a glance the range of choices you have. However, we don't mean to imply that these are the definitive ranges for each food category. For soups, for example, we have included primarily condensed canned soups made with water or milk, not restaurant soups, which are often higher in fat and energy density.

The first set of charts is organized according to the Food Guide Pyramid food groups. The second set includes beverages, mixed dishes, fast food, and desserts.

BREAD, CEREAL, RICE, AND PASTA GROUP

Our charts cover this food group in two sections: bread and grain products, and breakfast cereals.

Tips

- Select most often high-fiber whole grain complex carbohydrates, such as whole-wheat bread and brown rice.

- Cooked grains, even when they are refined, such as pasta, couscous, and white rice, are also good choices.

- White breads, including rolls and bagels, are slightly higher in energy density than whole grain versions or cooked grains.

- High-fiber breakfast cereals are often the lowest in energy density.

- Pay close attention to the serving sizes for this group. It's easy to eat portions that contain 3, 4, or more servings. Instead of a large bagel in the morning (4 servings), try half a bagel (2 servings) with low-fat yogurt and jam.

1. Bread and Grain Products. Note that cooked grains are lower in energy density than breads, and that reduced-fat crackers are still energy dense. (Grain data are based on cooked, not raw amounts.)

ENERGY DENSITY SPECTRUM

0.9 ———————————— 5.0

Bread and Grain Products	Serving Size	Calories	E.D. (cal/g)
Rice, Spanish	½ cup	108	0.9
Rice, wild, cooked	½ cup	83	1.0
Rice, long-grain, brown, cooked	½ cup	108	1.1
Couscous, cooked	½ cup	88	1.1
Rice, long-grain, white, cooked	½ cup	103	1.3
Pasta, noodles, egg, cooked	½ cup	106	1.3
Pasta, macaroni, cooked	½ cup	99	1.4
Pasta, spaghetti, cooked	½ cup	95	1.5
Rice, pilaf	½ cup	140	1.5
Tortilla, whole-wheat, fat-free	1 item (9″ diameter)	60	1.6
Stuffing, bread	½ cup	178	1.8
Stuffing, cornbread	½ cup	179	1.8
Bread, banana nut	1.4 oz. serving	246	2.0
Tortilla, corn	1 item (6″ diameter)	56	2.2
Pancakes, plain	1 item (7″ diameter)	166	2.3
French toast, prepared with 2 percent milk and margarine	1 slice	149	2.3
Bread, whole-wheat	1 slice	62	2.5
Waffle, plain, frozen	2 items (4½″ diameter)	191	2.5
English muffin	1 item	128	2.6
Bread, corn	1 slice	140	2.6
Bread, rye	1 slice	65	2.6

Bread and Grain Products	Serving Size	Calories	E.D. (cal/g)
Bread, pita, whole-wheat	1 item (6½" diameter)	170	2.7
Bread, white	1 slice	67	2.7
Bread, raisin	1 serving	106	2.7
Bread, Italian	1 slice (4½" x 3¼" x ¾")	81	2.7
Bagel, cinnamon raisin	1 item (3½" diameter)	195	2.7
Bread, French	1 slice (4¾" x 4" x ½")	69	2.7
Bread, sourdough	1 slice	69	2.7
Bagel, plain	1 item (3½" diameter)	195	2.8
Bread, pita, white	1 item (6½" diameter)	165	2.8
Muffin, bran	1 item (2¾" x 2")	161	2.8
Muffin, blueberry	1 item (2¾" x 2")	162	2.9
Bread, hamburger bun	1 item	123	2.9
Bread, hot dog bun	1 item	123	2.9
Waffle, plain, prepared	1 item (7" diameter)	218	2.9
Tortilla, flour	1 item (9" diameter)	114	3.3
Donut, jelly-filled	1 item (3½" x 2½")	289	3.4
Crackers, saltine, fat-free	10 items	100	3.6
Biscuit	1 item (2" x 1¼")	102	3.6
Cinnamon roll	1 item (3" diameter)	230	3.7
Bread, zucchini with nuts	1 slice	151	3.8
Melba toast	3 items	63	3.9
Toaster pastry, fruit	1 item	204	3.9
Matzo, plain	1 item (6" x 6")	112	4.0
Crackers, rye crisp bread	2 items	60	4.0

Bread and Grain Products	Serving Size	Calories	E.D. (cal/g)
Donut, glazed	1 item (3¼" diameter)	242	4.0
Crackers, Nabisco Triscuits, reduced fat	8 items	130	4.1
Croissant, butter	1 item	173	4.1
Pie crust	⅛ of 1 crust	110	4.1
Crackers, Wheat Thins, reduced fat	18 items	120	4.1
Donut, plain, old-fashioned	1 item (3" diameter)	198	4.2
Graham crackers	4 items (2½" x 2½")	118	4.2
Crackers, saltine	10 items	130	4.3
Crackers, Nabisco Triscuits, original	7 items	140	4.5
Crackers, wheat	10 items	142	4.7
Crackers, Wheat Thins, original	16 items	140	4.8
Crackers, cheese	30 items (1" x 1")	151	5.0

2. Breakfast Cereals. A cereal-based breakfast can be an excellent *Volumetric* way to start the day. You'll want to choose a high-fiber cereal, use low-fat or fat-free milk, and include fruit. Notice in this chart how much energy density goes down when you add low-fat milk. A half-cup of 1 percent low-fat milk adds about 50 calories.

Pay attention to volume, too. It is reflected in the serving size. Some puffed or flaked cereals take up a lot of room in your bowl, and that's important for satiety as well as weight. As snacks, dry cereal can be fairly high in energy density, so watch portions.

ENERGY DENSITY SPECTRUM

0.5———1.8

Breakfast Cereals	Serving Size	Calories	E.D.1/E.D.2* (cal/g)
Cream of wheat, regular, prepared with water, Nabisco	1 cup	121	0.6†/0.5
Farina (wheat), enriched, prepared with water and salt	1 cup	117	0.5†/0.5
Wheat and barley hot cereal, prepared with water	1 cup	122	0.5†/0.5
Oatmeal, prepared with water	1 cup	145	0.6†/0.6
Puffed Wheat Cereal, Quaker	1 cup	40	3.3/0.7
All-Bran Extra Fiber, Kellogg's	1 cup	100	1.7/0.8
Bran Flakes, Kellogg's	1 cup	98	3.3/1.0
Rice Chex, General Mills	1 cup	96	3.9/1.0
Toasties, Post	1 cup	100	3.6/1.0
Cheerios, General Mills	1 cup	110	3.7/1.1
Corn Chex, General Mills	1 cup	110	3.7/1.1
Corn Flakes, Kellogg's	1 cup	110	3.7/1.1
Product 19, Kellogg's	1 cup	110	3.7/1.1
Wheaties, General Mills	1 cup	110	3.7/1.1
Grape-Nuts Flakes Cereal, Post	1 cup	116	3.5/1.1
Crispix, Kellogg's	1 cup	115	3.6/1.1
Honey Nut Cheerios, General Mills	1 cup	120	4.0/1.1
All-Bran, Kellogg's	1 cup	165	2.5/1.2
Rice Krispies, Kellogg's	1 cup	138	3.7/1.2
Total, General Mills	1 cup	147	3.7/1.2
Smacks, Kellogg's	1 cup	147	3.7/1.2
Bran Flakes, Post	1 cup	154	3.3/1.2
Raisin Bran, Kellogg's	1 cup	170	3.1/1.3
Golden Crisp, Post	1 cup	147	4.1/1.3
Toasted Oatmeal, original, Quaker	1 cup	160	3.9/1.3
Honey Bunches of Oats, Post	1 cup	160	4.0/1.3
Shredded Wheat, Post	2 biscuits	170	3.6/1.3

*E.D.1 = dry cereal; E.D.2 = with 1/2 cup 1 percent milk

Breakfast Cereals	Serving Size	Calories	E.D.1/E.D.2* (cal/g)
Spoon Size Shredded Wheat, Post	1 cup	170	3.6/ 1.3
Raisin Bran, Post	1 cup	190	3.2/ 1.3
Bite Size Frosted Mini-Wheats, Kellogg's	1 cup	190	3.5/ 1.4
Multi Bran Chex, General Mills	1 cup	200	3.5/ 1.4
Shredded Wheat 'n Bran, Post	1 cup	198	3.6/ 1.4
100 Percent Bran, Post	1 cup	215	3.3/ 1.4
Shredded Wheat, Quaker	3 biscuits	220	3.5/ 1.5
Wheat Chex, General Mills	1 cup	240	3.6/ 1.5
Cracklin' Oat Bran, Kellogg's	1 cup	307	4.2/ 1.8
Grape-Nuts, Post	1 cup	400	3.5/ 1.9
Granola, reduced-fat, Healthy Choice	1 cup	380	3.9/ 2.0
100 percent Granola, Quaker	1 cup	440	4.6/ 2.3

*E.D.1 = dry cereal; E.D.2 = with 1/2 cup 1 percent milk

†Note: The energy density of hot cereals is for cooked cereal prepared with water; the information for serving with ½ cup milk refers to cooking the cereal with water and ½ cup of milk.

VEGETABLE GROUP

Tips

- Eat more! Vegetables, without added fat, have the lowest energy density of any food group.

- Most of the vegetables that fall into Category 1 are what nutritionists call nonstarchy vegetables. These include green vegetables, salad greens, tomatoes, green beans, summer squash, and onions. We encourage you to eat more of foods from this category. *Treat the recommendations as a minimum, with no maximum.*

- Most of the vegetables that fall into Category 2 are what nutritionists call starchy vegetables. These include potatoes, sweet potatoes, corn, dry beans, peas, lentils, and winter squash. These should also play a substantial role in your diet. But you can't eat them in unlimited quantities.

- Fried vegetables such as French fries or onion rings are in Categories 3 and 4; if you eat these, control portions carefully.

ENERGY DENSITY SPECTRUM

0.1 ——————————— 4.1

Vegetables	Serving Size	Calories	E.D. (cal/g)
Cucumbers, raw	1 cup	14	0.1
Lettuce, romaine	1 cup	8	0.1
Celery, raw	1 cup	19	0.2
Lettuce, loose leaf	1 cup	10	0.2
Bamboo shoots, canned	½ cup	12	0.2
Sauerkraut, canned	½ cup	22	0.2
Beans, green, canned, drained	½ cup	14	0.2
Squash, summer, boiled, drained	½ cup	18	0.2
Mung bean sprouts, boiled, drained	½ cup	13	0.2
Tomato, raw	1 item (medium)	26	0.2
Turnips, boiled, drained	½ cup	16	0.2
Tomatoes, diced, canned	½ cup	25	0.2
Spinach, chopped	1 cup	7	0.2
Cauliflower, boiled, drained	½ cup	14	0.2
Asparagus, boiled, drained	½ cup	22	0.2
Tomatoes, whole, canned	½ cup	25	0.2
Cabbage, raw	1 cup	18	0.3
Cauliflower, raw	½ cup	13	0.3
Mushrooms, raw	½ cup	9	0.3
Collard greens, boiled, drained	½ cup	25	0.3
Mushrooms, boiled, drained	½ cup	21	0.3
Peppers, green, raw	½ cup	20	0.3
Beans, green, frozen, boiled, drained	½ cup	19	0.3
Broccoli, boiled, drained	½ cup	22	0.3

Vegetables	Serving Size	Calories	E.D. (cal/g)
Eggplant, boiled, drained	½ cup	13	0.3
Broccoli, raw	½ cup	12	0.3
Alfalfa sprouts	¼ cup	2	0.3
Leeks, boiled, drained	½ cup	16	0.3
Fennel bulb, boiled, drained	1 item (medium)	73	0.3
Okra, boiled, drained	½ cup	26	0.3
Pumpkin, canned	½ cup	42	0.3
Beans, green, boiled, drained	½ cup	22	0.3
Onions, raw	¼ cup	15	0.4
Brussels sprouts, boiled, drained	½ cup	30	0.4
Squash, winter, baked	½ cup	40	0.4
Carrots, raw	1 cup	52	0.4
Beets, boiled, drained	½ cup	37	0.4
Onions, chopped, boiled, drained	½ cup	46	0.4
Carrots, sliced, boiled, drained	½ cup	35	0.5
Water chestnuts, canned	½ cup	35	0.5
Green peas, frozen, boiled, drained	½ cup	62	0.8
Parsnips, boiled, drained	½ cup	63	0.8
Corn, canned, boiled, drained	½ cup	66	0.8
Green peas, raw	½ cup	59	0.8
Potatoes, scalloped	½ cup	105	0.9
Corn on the cob, boiled, drained	1 item (medium)	77	0.9
Sweet potato, baked	½ cup	103	1.0
Potatoes, mashed with margarine and whole milk	½ cup	111	1.1
Potato, baked with skin	1 item (medium)	220	1.1
Potatoes, hash browned	½ cup	163	2.1
Potatoes, French-fried	1 ounce	91	3.2
Onions, batter-dipped and fried, frozen	7 items (medium)	285	4.1

FRUIT GROUP

Tips

- Most whole fresh fruits are in Category 1, and we encourage you to eat more of them. *Use the serving recommendations above as a minimum, with no maximum.*

- Fruits canned in syrup are in Category 2. Enjoy these but pay attention to portion sizes. Look for fruits canned in light syrup or in their natural juices rather than in heavy syrup.

- Dried fruits are in Category 3. They are quite energy dense. They are healthy alternatives to candy bars, but keep portions small: ¼ cup or less.

- Fruit juices are listed in the "Beverages" chart (p. 133).

ENERGY DENSITY SPECTRUM

0.2 —————— 3.0

Fruit	Serving Size	Calories	E.D (cal/g)
Strawberries	½ cup	18	0.2
Grapefruit, pink and red	½ item (medium)	37	0.3
Raspberries	½ cup	18	0.3
Watermelon, diced	1 cup	49	0.3
Cantaloupe, cubed	1 cup	56	0.4
Honeydew, cubed	1 cup	62	0.4
Papaya	½ cup	27	0.4
Peaches, canned in light syrup	½ cup	52	0.4
Applesauce, unsweetened	½ cup	52	0.4
Peach	1 item (medium)	42	0.4
Tangerine	2 items (medium)	74	0.4
Orange	1 item (medium)	62	0.5

Fruit	Serving Size	Calories	E.D (cal/g)
Apricot	4 items (medium)	67	0.5
Pears, canned in light syrup	½ cup	60	0.5
Pineapple	½ cup	38	0.5
Pineapple, canned in light syrup	½ cup	66	0.5
Plum	1 item (medium)	36	0.6
Blueberries	½ cup	40	0.6
Fruit cocktail, canned in light syrup	½ cup	69	0.6
Apple	1 item (medium)	81	0.6
Pear	1 item (medium)	98	0.6
Mandarin oranges, canned in light syrup	½ cup	77	0.6
Mango	½ cup	54	0.7
Grapes	1½ cup	92	0.7
Kiwi fruit, peeled	1 item (medium)	53	0.7
Pears, canned in heavy syrup	½ cup	90	0.7
Cherries, sweet	½ cup	52	0.7
Fruit cocktail, canned in heavy syrup	½ cup	91	0.7
Peaches, canned in heavy syrup	½ cup	128	0.9
Banana	1 item (medium)	109	0.9
Apricots, dried	¼ cup	77	2.4
Prunes, dried	¼ cup	102	2.4
Dates	¼ cup	122	2.7
Raisins	¼ cup	109	3.0

MILK, YOGURT, AND CHEESE GROUP

Tips

- This category varies in energy density by tenfold! Low-fat or fat-free milk, yogurt, cottage cheese, and sour cream are low in energy density. Portion control is important with low-fat hard cheeses, and becomes essential with full-fat hard cheeses, which are very energy dense.

- Low-fat (1 percent) or fat-free milk is in Category 1. So is nonfat yogurt. These are excellent choices.

- Low-fat cottage cheese and low-fat sour cream are in Category 2. So are fat-free versions of these foods. They are all good choices.

- Low-fat frozen yogurt, low-fat ice cream, and ice milk are low in energy density when compared with other dessert choices.

- Hard cheeses such as cheddar, even those that are reduced in fat, are still fairly high in energy density. Use these in moderation. However, intensely flavored energy-dense grating cheeses like Parmesan can be used in small amounts to add flavor to foods with few calories.

ENERGY DENSITY SPECTRUM

0.4 ——————— 4.0

Milk, Yogurt and Cheese	Serving Size	Calories	E.D. (cal/g)
Milk, nonfat/skim	8 fluid oz.	86	0.4
Milk, low-fat (1 percent)	8 fluid oz.	102	0.4
Milk, reduced fat (2 percent)	8 fluid oz.	121	0.5
Yogurt, sugar-free low-fat (1 percent) fruit-flavored	6 oz.	90	0.5
Yogurt, fat-free, plain	1 cup	137	0.6
Milk, whole (3.3 percent)	8 fluid oz.	150	0.6
Cottage cheese, fat-free	½ cup	80	0.7
Milk, reduced-fat (2 percent), chocolate	8 fluid oz.	179	0.7

Milk, Yogurt and Cheese	Serving Size	Calories	E.D. (cal/g)
Milk, whole, chocolate	8 fluid oz.	208	0.8
Cottage cheese, reduced-fat (2 percent)	½ cup	101	0.9
Sour cream, fat-free	2 tablespoons	30	0.9
Yogurt, fruit-flavors, 99 percent fat-free	6 oz.	170	1.0
Cottage cheese, full-fat (4 percent)	½ cup	109	1.0
Cream cheese, fat-free	2 tablespoons	30	1.1
Yogurt, frozen, fat-free, vanilla	½ cup	80	1.2
Yogurt, frozen, fruit flavors	½ cup	144	1.3
Cream, half and half	2 tablespoons	39	1.3
Ice cream, light, vanilla	½ cup	92	1.4
Sour cream, reduced fat	2 tablespoons	45	1.5
Cream, light	2 tablespoons	59	2.0
Sour cream, full-fat	2 tablespoons	60	2.0
Cream cheese, reduced-fat	2 tablespoons	70	2.5
Ice cream, premium, vanilla/chocolate	½ cup	270	2.6
Cheese, mozzarella, part skim	1 ounce	73	2.6
Cheese, feta	1 ounce	74	2.6
Cheese, mozzarella, whole milk	1 ounce	79	2.8
Cheese, cheddar, reduced-fat	1 ounce	90	3.2
Cheese, provolone	1 ounce	98	3.5
Cream cheese, full-fat	2 tablespoons	100	3.5
Cheese, blue	1 ounce	100	3.5
Cheese, American	1 ounce	106	3.8
Cheese, Swiss	1 ounce	105	3.8
Cheese, cheddar	1 ounce	110	3.9
Cheese, Parmesan, grated	2 teaspoons	20	4.0
Cheese, Parmesan, grated, fat-free	2 teaspoons	20	4.0

MEAT, POULTRY, FISH, LEGUMES, EGGS, AND NUTS GROUP

We cover this food group in 4 charts: legumes; meat, poultry, and fish; eggs; and nuts and seeds.

Tips

- Legumes, such as navy or pinto beans, have the lowest energy density for protein foods. They are at the lowest end of Category 2.

- Lean fish and most seafood are at the lower end of Category 2. Even fattier fish like tuna and salmon, with beneficial fish oils, are still in Category 2. These are excellent choices.

- Lean poultry, veal, and extra lean ham are also in Category 2.

- Egg substitutes are at the lower end of Category 2, while whole eggs cooked without added fat (for instance, soft boiled) are at the upper end of Category 2. Fried eggs are in Category 3.

- Lean beef and pork, trimmed of fat, are at the lower end of Category 3. Sirloin steak, for instance, is lower in energy density than hamburger.

- Frying boosts energy density so much that fried fish is much higher in energy density that broiled sirloin steak.

- Nuts and seeds are very high in energy density: Category 4. Use these in small amounts. If you are a vegetarian, however, you may want to include 2–4 tablespoons per person as a protein source in dishes that contain lower-energy-dense whole grains and vegetables.

- Pay attention to portion size for protein-rich foods. They are often served in supersize portions. It's fine if you want a 6-ounce serving of broiled chicken breast without the skin for dinner; just remember to count it as 2 servings. Try mixed dishes, including casseroles and stir-fries, that use 2–3 ounces of lean meat, poultry, or fish per person with plenty of vegetables.

1. Legumes. Dry beans, peas, chickpeas, lentils, and soy foods like tofu are nutritious protein sources. They're also rich in many vitamins and minerals, as well as fiber. Tofu, which contains a good amount of water, is almost in Category 1! The rest are in Category 2, except for hummus, which has added fat and is in a lower rung of Category 3.

ENERGY DENSITY SPECTRUM

0.6 ——— 1.7

Legumes	Serving Size	Calories	E.D. (cal/g)
Tofu, raw, soft	4 oz.	69	0.6
Beans, black, canned	½ cup	100	0.8
Beans, kidney, canned	½ cup	104	0.8
Beans, baked, canned	½ cup	118	0.9
Beans, refried, fat-free, canned	½ cup	123	1.0
Beans, refried, canned	½ cup	125	1.0
Lentils, boiled	½ cup	115	1.2
Split peas, boiled	½ cup	116	1.2
Chickpeas (garbanzo beans), canned	½ cup	143	1.2
Beans, lima, boiled, drained	½ cup	105	1.2
Beans, navy, boiled	½ cup	129	1.4
Hummus	½ cup	210	1.7

2. Meat, Poultry, and Fish. Lean selections from this group, cooked with little added fat, are excellent choices. They fall into either Category 2 or the lower rungs of Category 3. Fish, even fattier fish such as salmon, are particularly good low-density choices.

ENERGY DENSITY SPECTRUM

0.9 ——————————— 5.0

Meat, Poultry and Fish	Serving Size	Calories	E.D. (cal/g)
Orange roughy, cooked, dry heat	3 oz.	76	0.9
Shrimp, boiled or steamed	3 oz.	84	1.0
Tuna, canned in water	2 oz.	60	1.1

Meat, Poultry and Fish	Serving Size	Calories	E.D. (cal/g)
Veal chop, braised	3 oz.	99	1.2
Perch, cooked, dry heat	3 oz.	99	1.2
Turkey tenderloin	3 oz.	110	1.3
Ham, extra lean, 5 percent fat	3 oz.	111	1.3
Yellowfin tuna, cooked, dry heat	3 oz.	118	1.4
Halibut, cooked, dry heat	3 oz.	119	1.4
Turkey, breast, ground, 99 percent fat-free	3 oz.	120	1.4
Salmon, pink, cooked, dry heat	3 oz.	127	1.5
Chicken liver, simmered	3 oz.	133	1.6
Turkey breast, roasted, no skin	3 oz.	133	1.6
Chicken breast, roasted, no skin	3 oz.	140	1.7
Swordfish, broiled with margarine	3 oz.	151	1.8
Ham, 11 percent fat	3 oz.	155	1.8
Sirloin steak, lean, broiled	3 oz.	158	1.9
Turkey, ground, lean 7 percent fat	3 oz.	160	1.9
Tuna, canned in oil	2 oz.	110	2.0
Chicken breast, roasted	3 oz.	167	2.0
Pork chop, center loin, broiled	3 oz.	172	2.0
Chicken breast, fried	3 oz.	189	2.2
Fish, battered and fried	3 oz.	198	2.3
Bologna, pork	2 slices (4" diameter x ⅛" thick)	114	2.5
Lamb leg, whole, choice, ¼" fat	3 oz.	219	2.6
Salami, beef, cooked	2 slices (4" diameter x ½" thick)	121	2.6
Bratwurst	1 item (6")	240	2.6

Meat, Poultry and Fish	Serving Size	Calories	E.D. (cal/g)
Chicken, pieces, boneless, breaded and fried	6 pieces	287	2.7
Ground beef, lean, broiled, medium	3 oz.	231	2.7
Beef jerky	1 ounce	80	2.9
Chicken wing, meat and skin, roasted	3 oz.	247	2.9
Bologna, beef	2 slices (4½" diameter x ⅛" thick)	177	3.1
Frankfurter, beef	1 item (5" x ¾")	142	3.2
Italian sausage (pork),	3 oz. cooked	275	3.2
Bacon	2 slices	70	5.0
pork rinds, fried	1 ounce	155	5.5

3. Eggs. Eggs and egg substitutes, cooked with little added fat, are good protein choices.

ENERGY DENSITY SPECTRUM

0.8 —— 2.0

Egg	Serving Size	Calories	E.D. (cal/g)
Egg substitute, liquid	½ cup	106	0.9
Egg, poached	1 item (large)	75	1.5
Egg, hard-boiled	1 item (large)	78	1.6
Egg, scrambled with milk and butter	½ cup	183	1.6
Egg, fried	1 item (large)	92	2.0

4. Nuts and Seeds. These are highly nutritious but also very energy dense.

ENERGY DENSITY SPECTRUM

5.7 — 6.6

Nuts	Serving Size	Calories	E.D. (cal/g)
Sesame seeds, roasted, toasted	¼ cup	204	5.7
Cashews, dry roasted	¼ cup	197	5.7
Sunflower seeds, roasted	¼ cup	186	5.8
Peanuts, dry roasted	¼ cup	214	5.9
Almonds, dry roasted, unblanched, salted	¼ cup	203	5.9
Pecans, dry roasted, salted	¼ cup	178	6.6

BEVERAGES AND MIXED FOODS

THE USDA FOOD GUIDE PYRAMID gives advice on single foods, but most of the foods we eat are in mixed meals. Here we provide you with the energy density spectrum of some common foods and drinks.

BEVERAGES

Because thirst is regulated differently from hunger, the energy density of beverages should be used to compare drinks with one another, not with foods. Thus, soft drinks or beers, with "low" energy densities of only 0.4, can add hundreds of hidden calories to your diet. Hard alcohol and mixed drinks are even more energy dense. Low E.D. choices: water, diet soda, tea or coffee, nonalcoholic beer, vegetable juice, or sugar-free hot chocolate.

ENERGY DENSITY SPECTRUM

0 —————————— 3.7

Beverages	Serving Size	Calories	E.D. (cal/g)
Club soda	12 fluid oz.	0	0.0
Soda, lemon-lime, diet	12 fluid oz.	0	0.0
Tap water	8 fluid oz.	0	0.0
Tea, iced, unsweetened, with lemon	12 fluid oz.	0	0.0
Cola, diet	12 fluid oz.	2	0.0

Beverages	Serving Size	Calories	E.D. (cal/g)
Root beer, diet	12 fluid oz.	2	0.0
Soda, orange, diet	12 fluid oz.	3	0.1
Tea, brewed, without sugar	8 fluid oz.	2	0.1
Coffee	8 fluid oz.	5	0.2
Coffee with 1 teaspoon cream and 1 teaspoon sugar	12 fluid oz.	32	0.1
Beer, nonalcoholic	12 fluid oz.	32	0.1
Sports beverage	8 fluid oz.	50	0.2
Vegetable juice	8 fluid oz.	50	0.2
Cocoa, hot, from sugar-free cocoa mix, prepared with water	8 fluid oz.	64	0.3
Beer, light	12 fluid oz.	99	0.3
Milk, soy, plain	8 fluid oz.	79	0.3
Tea, iced, presweetened, with lemon	12 fluid oz.	120	0.3
Ginger ale	12 fluid oz.	124	0.3
Fruit punch	8 fluid oz.	97	0.4
Grapefruit juice	8 fluid oz.	96	0.4
Apple cider, fermented	4 fluid oz.	47	0.4
Carrot juice	8 fluid oz.	98	0.4
Lemonade	8 fluid oz.	99	0.4
Soda, lemon-lime	12 fluid oz.	147	0.4
Cola	12 fluid oz.	152	0.4
Root beer	12 fluid oz.	152	0.4
Beer	12 fluid oz.	146	0.4
Orange juice	8 fluid oz.	112	0.5
Pineapple juice	8 fluid oz.	110	0.5
Apple juice	8 fluid oz.	117	0.5
Soda, orange	12 fluid oz.	179	0.5
Cocoa, hot, from cocoa mix, prepared with water	8 fluid oz.	124	0.5
Wine cooler	8 fluid oz.	120	0.5
Soda, cream	12 fluid oz.	189	0.5
Cranberry juice cocktail	8 fluid oz.	144	0.6

Beverages	Serving Size	Calories	E.D. (cal/g)
Grape juice	8 fluid oz.	154	0.6
Malt drink, prepared from mix with whole milk	8 fluid oz.	170	0.6
Wine, white	4 fluid oz.	80	0.7
Champagne	4 fluid oz.	84	0.7
Gin and tonic	7.1 fluid oz.	151	0.7
Wine, red	4 fluid oz.	85	0.7
Eggnog	8 fluid oz.	342	1.4
Sherry, dry	4 fluid oz.	168	1.4
Pina colada	4½ fluid oz.	262	1.9
Daiquiri	4 fluid oz.	225	1.9
Margarita	4 fluid oz.	271	2.2
Distilled alcohol (80 proof)	1 fluid oz.	64	2.3
Gin	1 fluid ounce	64	2.3
Cognac	1 fluid ounce	73	2.4
Whiskey	1 fluid ounce	73	2.6
Distilled alcohol (100 proof)	1 fluid ounce	82	3.0
Creme de menthe (72 proof)	1 fluid ounce	125	3.7

SOUPS

You already know how *Volumetric* soups can be, but they do vary in energy density. You'll get less than half the calories from a cup of vegetable beef soup than from a cup of cream of mushroom soup made with 2 percent reduced-fat milk.

ENERGY DENSITY SPECTRUM

0.1–0.8

Soups	Serving Size	Calories	E.D. (cal/g)
Chicken broth, fat-free	1 cup	15	0.1
Beef broth	1 cup	30	0.1
Chicken broth	1 cup	39	0.2
Gazpacho soup, canned	1 cup	46	0.2

Soups	Serving Size	Calories	E.D. (cal/g)
Onion soup, condensed, canned, prepared with water	1 cup	58	0.2
Vegetarian vegetable soup	1 cup	72	0.3
Chicken noodle soup, condensed, canned, prepared with water	1 cup	75	0.3
Minestrone soup, condensed, canned, prepared with water	1 cup	82	0.3
Vegetable beef soup	1 cup	82	0.3
Tomato soup, condensed, canned, prepared with water	1 cup	85	0.4
New England clam chowder, condensed, canned, prepared with water	1 cup	95	0.4
Chicken, rice, and vegetable soup	1 cup	110	0.5
Black bean soup, condensed, canned, prepared with water	1 cup	116	0.5
Lentil and ham soup, canned	1 cup	139	0.6
Tomato soup, condensed, canned, prepared with 2 percent milk	1 cup	161	0.7
Split pea soup with ham	1 cup	160	0.7
Cream of broccoli with cheese soup	1 cup	190	0.8
Cream of mushroom soup, condensed, canned, prepared with 2 percent milk	1 cup	203	0.8

CHIPS, PRETZELS, AND OTHER SNACK FOODS

Low-fat and fat-free chips are lower in energy density than regular
full-fat ones, but still fairly energy dense.

ENERGY DENSITY SPECTRUM

2.5 ——————— 5.4

Chips, Pretzels, and Other Snack Foods	Serving Size	Calories	E.D. (cal/g)
Pretzel, soft	1 item (3 oz.)	210	2.5
Chips, potato, fat-free	1 ounce	75	2.7
Chips, tortilla, white corn, fat-free (with olestra)	1 ounce (6 large chips)	90	3.2
Pretzels, hard, salted	1 ounce	108	3.8
Popcorn, plain, popped	3 cups	92	3.8
Rice cakes, plain	3 items	104	3.9
Chips, tortilla, white corn, low-fat (baked)	1 ounce (9 medium chips)	110	3.9
Chips, potato, baked	1 ounce	113	4.0
Popcorn, caramel	1 cup	152	4.3
Trail mix	¼ cup	173	4.6
Chips, tortilla, white corn	1 ounce (6 large chips)	130	4.6
Popcorn, popped in oil	3 cups	135	5.0
Cheese puffs	15 items (1 ounce)	150	5.4
Chips, potato, regular	1 ounce	150	5.4
Chips, corn	1 ounce	153	5.4

MIXED FOODS

Lower energy-dense choices include vegetarian three-bean chili, beef
stew with vegetables, tuna and noodles, and chicken chow mein.

ENERGY DENSITY SPECTRUM

0.7 ——————— 3.2

Mixed Foods	Serving Size	Calories	E.D. (cal/g)
Chili, vegetarian with three beans	1 cup	160	0.7
Cole slaw	½ cup	41	0.7
Three-bean salad	1 serving	48	0.9
Beef stew with vegetables	1 cup	220	0.9
Tuna and noodles	1 serving	254	1.0
Pasta salad, packaged	¾ cup	250	1.0
Chicken chow mein	1 cup	255	1.0
Chili with beans, canned	½ cup	143	1.1
Potato salad	½ cup	134	1.1
Pork and beans, canned	½ cup	157	1.2
Chop suey with beef and pork	1 cup	300	1.2
Chili con carne with beans, canned	1 cup	322	1.3
Spaghetti with meat sauce	¾ cup	320	1.5
Macaroni salad	½ cup	134	1.5
Lasagna with meat	1 piece (3½" x 4")	370	1.6
Vegetable burger	1 item	130	1.8
Tuna salad	½ cup	192	1.9
Meat loaf	1 serving (4⅓ oz.)	232	1.9
Bean and cheese burrito	1 item	189	2.0
Fettuccini Alfredo, frozen	10 oz.	580	2.0
Chicken pot pie, frozen	1 item	410	2.1
Taco	1 item	369	2.2
Chicken salad	½ cup	209	2.3
Carrot and raisin salad	½ cup	210	2.4
Macaroni and cheese	¾ cup	355	2.5
Hot dog with bun, plain	1 item	242	2.5
Pizza, thin crust, sausage, frozen	½ pizza	380	2.5
Nachos with beef, beans, cheese, tomatoes, and onions	1 serving	394	2.7

Mixed Foods	Serving Size	Calories	E.D. (cal/g)
Cheese pizza, thick crust	1 slice (⅛ of 12" diameter)	202	2.9
Pizza, thin crust, pepperoni	¼ pizza	400	2.9
Ravioli, cheese, refrigerated	1 cup	280	3.2

FAST FOODS

Can you eat on the run and still follow a *Volumetric* way of eating? Sure, if you choose carefully. A Subway turkey breast sandwich made without oil or mayo has an E.D. of only 1.2, which means you get only 290 calories in a big sandwich. But one large piece of KFC's Hot and Spicy Chicken breast (E.D.: 2.9) gives you 530 calories. A better choice within that restaurant: Tender Roast Chicken breast without the skin (E.D.: 1.4; calories: 170).

ENERGY DENSITY SPECTRUM

0.4 —————————— 4.2

Fast Foods	Serving Size	Calories	E.D. (cal/g)
Little Caesar's, Crazy Sauce	1 packet (6.0 oz.)	74	0.4
Church's Chicken, potatoes and gravy	1 order (3.7 oz.)	90	0.9
Wendy's, chili, small	8.0 oz.	210	0.9
Hardee's, vanilla shake	12.3 oz.	350	1.0
Arby's, barbecue sauce	0.5 oz.	15	1.1
Subway, turkey breast sandwich with lettuce, tomatoes, onions, pickles, green peppers, and olives on wheat bread	1 sandwich (6")	289	1.2
KFC, Tender Roast Chicken breast (without skin)	1 piece (4.2 oz.)	169	1.4

Fast Foods	Serving Size	Calories	E.D. (cal/g)
Subway, cold cut trio sandwich with lettuce, tomatoes, onions, pickles, green peppers, and olives on white bread	1 sandwich (6")	362	1.5
Subway, tuna sandwich with lettuce, tomatoes, onions, pickles, green peppers, and olives on wheat bread	1 sandwich (6")	391	1.6
Taco Bell, taco salad with salsa	1 salad (19.0 oz.)	850	1.6
Taco Bell, Big Beef Burrito Supreme	1 burrito (10.5 oz.)	520	1.8
KFC, Tender Roast Chicken breast (with skin)	1 piece (4.9 oz.)	251	1.8
Wendy's, hamburger, single with everything	1 sandwich (7.7 oz.)	420	1.9
Long John Silver's, fish, batter-dipped	1 piece (3.0 oz.)	170	2.0
Taco Bell, Steak Fajita Wrap	1 wrap (8.0 oz.)	470	2.1
Pizza Hut, Thin 'N Crispy Pizza, Veggie Lover's	1 slice med. pizza	222	2.1
Wendy's, chicken sandwich, breaded, with mayonnaise	1 sandwich (7.3 oz.)	440	2.1
Hardee's, cole slaw	1 order (4.0 oz.)	240	2.1
McDonald's, Egg McMuffin	1 item	290	2.1
Burger King, Broiler chicken sandwich with mayonnaise	1 sandwich	530	2.2
Taco Bell, taco	1 taco (2.8 oz.)	180	2.3
McDonald's, Fish Filet Deluxe with tartar sauce and cheese	1 sandwich	560	2.5

Fast Foods	Serving Size	Calories	E.D. (cal/g)
Church's Chicken, chicken leg	1 piece (2.0 oz.)	140	2.5
Taco Bell, Nachos BellGrande	1 order (11.0 oz.)	770	2.5
Church's Chicken, chicken breast	1 piece (2.8 oz.)	200	2.5
Arby's, roast beef sandwich, regular	1 sandwich	388	2.5
Arby's, Beef 'n Cheddar Sandwich	1 sandwich (6.7 oz.)	487	2.6
Burger King, Whopper with cheese and mayonnaise	1 sandwich	760	2.6
McDonald's, Big Mac	1 sandwich	560	2.6
Hardee's, cheeseburger	1 sandwich	320	2.6
KFC, Original Recipe Chicken breast	1 piece (5.4 oz.)	400	2.6
McDonald's, Quarter Pounder with Cheese, no mayonnaise	1 sandwich	530	2.7
Little Caesar's, Crazy Bread	1 piece (1.4 oz.)	106	2.7
McDonald's, Chicken McNuggets	4 pieces	190	2.7
Pizza Hut, Hand Tossed Pizza, Super Supreme	1 slice medium pizza	359	2.7
Jack in the Box, double cheeseburger	1 sandwich	460	2.8
KFC, Extra Tasty Crispy Chicken breast	1 piece (5.9 oz.)	470	2.8
KFC, Hot and Spicy Chicken breast	1 piece (6.5 oz.)	530	3.0
Wendy's, French fries, small order	1 order (3.2 oz.)	270	3.0
Pizza Hut, Hand Tossed Pizza, cheese	1 slice medium pizza	309	3.0
Hardee's, French fries	1 order (regular; 3.4 oz.)	340	3.0

Fast Foods	Serving Size	Calories	E.D. (cal/g)
McDonald's, French fries	1 order (small; 2.4 oz.)	210	3.1
Jack in the Box, seasoned curly fries	1 order (4.5 oz.)	410	3.3
Pizza Hut, pan pizza, pepperoni	1 slice med. pizza	353	3.3
McDonald's, apple pie, baked	1 item	260	3.4
Arby's, French fries	1 order (2.5 oz.)	246	3.5
McDonald's, bacon, egg, and cheese biscuit	1 item	547	3.5
Burger King, Croissan'wich with sausage, egg, and cheese	1 item	530	3.5
Dunkin' Donuts, glazed donut	1 item (1.6 oz.)	160	3.5
Dunkin' Donuts, jelly-filled donut	1 item (2.4 oz.)	240	3.5
Burger King, French Toast Sticks	1 order (5 items)	440	3.9
Burger King, onion rings	1 order (medium)	380	4.0
Arby's, Horsey Sauce	0.5 ounce	60	4.2

CONDIMENTS, DRESSINGS, AND SAUCES

What you spread on your bread, what you use to make your sandwich, and what you toss with your salad vary enormously in energy density. If you dip veggies into salsa (E.D.: 0.3) rather than full-fat ranch dressing (E.D.: 4.0), you'll reduce the calories by 90 percent!

ENERGY DENSITY SPECTRUM

0.1 ————————————————————————— 8.9

Condiments, Dressing, and Sauces	Serving Size	Calories	E.D. (cal/g)
Vinegar	1 tablespoon	2	0.1
Pickles, dill	1 item, 3¾″ long	12	0.2
Lemon juice	1 tablespoon	4	0.3
Salsa	2 tablespoons	4	0.3
Dressing, Italian, fat-free	2 tablespoons	15	0.5
Gravy, turkey	2 oz.	29	0.5
Syrup, maple-flavored, sugar-free	¼ cup	30	0.5
Soy sauce	1 tablespoon	10	0.5
Preserves, apricot, sugar-free	1 tablespoon	10	0.6
Preserves, strawberry, sugar-free	1 tablespoon	10	0.6
Mayonnaise, fat-free	1 tablespoon	10	0.6
Worcestershire sauce	1 teaspoon	4	0.7
Barbecue sauce	2 tablespoons	23	0.8
Horseradish	1 teaspoon	4	0.9
Cocktail sauce	1 tablespoon	15	0.9
Ketchup	1 tablespoon	15	0.9
Mustard, yellow	1 teaspoon	5	1.0
Relish, pickle	1 tablespoon	15	1.0
Dressing, French, fat-free	2 tablespoons	35	1.0
Spaghetti sauce	½ cup	140	1.1
Pickles, sweet, gherkin	1 item (2½″)	18	1.2
Dressing, thousand island, fat-free	2 tablespoons	40	1.2
Dressing, blue cheese, fat-free	2 tablespoons	50	1.4
Dressing, ranch, fat-free	2 tablespoons	50	1.4
Preserves, strawberry, reduced-sugar	1 tablespoon	25	1.5
Dressing, Italian, reduced-fat	2 tablespoons	50	1.6
Olives, black, canned	6 items	25	1.7
Olives, green, canned	7 items	25	1.7
Whipped topping, frozen, fat-free	2 tablespoons	15	1.7

Condiments, Dressing, and Sauces	Serving Size	Calories	E.D. (cal/g)
Syrup, maple-flavored, reduced-calorie	¼ cup	100	1.7
Apple butter	1 tablespoon	30	1.8
Margarine, low-calorie	1 tablespoon	30	2.1
Dressing, thousand island, reduced-fat	2 tablespoons	70	2.2
Whipped topping, frozen, reduced-fat	2 tablespoons	20	2.2
Pesto sauce, frozen	1 ounce	66	2.3
Jelly, grape	1 tablespoon	50	2.5
Marmalade, orange	1 tablespoon	50	2.5
Preserves, apricot	1 tablespoon	50	2.5
Preserves, red raspberry	1 tablespoon	50	2.5
Preserves, strawberry	1 tablespoon	50	2.5
Chocolate syrup	2 tablespoons	102	2.6
Dressing, ranch, reduced-fat	2 tablespoons	80	2.7
Whipped topping, frozen, regular	2 tablespoons	25	2.8
Honey	1 tablespoon	60	2.9
Mayonnaise, light	1 tablespoon	50	3.3
Marshmallow cream topping	2 tablespoons	40	3.3
Fudge topping	2 tablespoons	130	3.4
Dressing, Italian, full-fat	2 tablespoons	110	3.6
Dressing, thousand island, full-fat	2 tablespoons	110	3.6
Butter, light	1 tablespoon	50	3.6
Syrup, maple-flavored	¼ cup	210	3.6
Dressing, French, full-fat	2 tablespoons	120	3.8
Dressing, blue cheese, full-fat	2 tablespoons	120	4.0
Tartar sauce	1 tablespoon	72	5.2
Peanut butter, reduced-fat	2 tablespoons	190	5.3
Dressing, ranch, full-fat	2 tablespoons	170	5.9
Peanut butter	2 tablespoons	190	5.9
Butter, whipped	1 tablespoon	60	6.7
Mayonnaise, full-fat	1 tablespoon	100	7.2

Condiments, Dressing, and Sauces	Serving Size	Calories	E.D. (cal/g)
Butter	1 tablespoon	108	7.2
Margarine	1 tablespoon	101	7.2
Oil, vegetable	1 tablespoon	120	8.8

DESSERTS

Lower energy-dense choices in this category include gelatin desserts, baked fruit, Italian ice, sorbet, sherbet, pudding, frozen fruit bars, and fat-free fudge bars.

ENERGY DENSITY SPECTRUM

0.1 ———————————————5.0

Desserts	Serving Size	Calories	E.D. (cal/g)
Gelatin, fruit-flavored, sugar-free	½ cup	10	0.1
Gelatin, fruit-flavored	½ cup	80	0.6
Apple, baked, unsweetened	1 item (medium)	102	0.6
Italian ice, lemon	1 item (8 oz.)	140	0.8
Fruit and juice bar, frozen	1 item (3 oz.)	75	0.8
Fruit-flavored frozen pop	1 item	45	0.9
Vanilla pudding, prepared with 2 percent milk	½ cup	141	1.0
Chocolate pudding, prepared with 2 percent milk	½ cup	151	1.1
Sherbet, all flavors	½ cup	133	1.4
Fudge bar, frozen	1 item (2.5 oz.)	104	1.4
Pudding, rice	½ cup	175	1.6
Pumpkin pie	⅛ of 8″ pie	229	2.1
Peach pie	⅙ of 8″ pie	261	2.2
Apple pie	⅛ of 9″ pie	296	2.4

Desserts	Serving Size	Calories	E.D. (cal/g)
Coffee cake, cinnamon apple, fat-free	1/9 of 17 oz. cake	130	2.4
Angel food cake	1/12 of 10" cake	129	2.6
Cherry pie	1/8 of 9" pie	325	2.6
Banana cream pie	1/8 of 9" pie	398	2.7
Fruit chewy cookies (Fig Newtons) fat-free	2 items	90	3.1
Cheesecake	1/6 of 17 oz. cake	257	3.2
Fruit chewy cookies (Fig Newtons)	2 items	110	3.6
Chocolate cupcake, cream-filled	2 items	230	3.59
Chocolate cake with frosting	1/2 of 9" layer cake	235	3.67
Ice cream, cake cone	1 item	30	3.8
White cake with frosting	1/2 of 9" layer cake	252	3.8
Pound cake, ready-to-eat	1/10 of 12 oz. cake	116	3.9
Granola bar, chewy, chocolate chip, low-fat	1 item	110	3.9
Frosting, chocolate, homemade	2 tablespoons	193	3.9
Frosting, chocolate, ready-to-eat	2 tablespoons	130	3.9
Frosting, white, homemade	2 tablespoons	163	4.1
Frosting, white, ready-to-eat	2 tablespoons	140	4.1
Coffee cake with crumb topping	1/9 of 20 oz. cake	263	4.2
Graham crackers	4 items (2½" x 2½")	118	4.2
Granola bar, chewy, chocolate chip	1 item	120	4.3
Granola bar, oats and honey	2 items	180	4.3

Desserts	Serving Size	Calories	E.D. (cal/g)
Carrot cake with cream cheese frosting	1/12 of 9" cake	484	4.4
Vanilla wafers	8 items	140	4.4
Creme-filled sandwich cookies, reduced-fat	2 items	130	4.5
Chocolate chip cookies, reduced-fat	3 items	140	4.5
Peanut butter cookies, homemade	2 items	165	4.6
Chocolate chip cookies, homemade	2 items	143	4.6
Brownie, ready-to-eat	1 item (2" x 2")	112	4.7
Animal crackers	10 items	140	4.7
Creme-filled sandwich cookies	2 items	140	4.8
Chocolate creme-filled sandwich cookies	3 items	160	4.9
Chocolate chip cookies	3 items	160	5.0
Shortbread cookies	3 items	160	5.0

CANDIES

Even fat-free or low-fat candies (marshmallows, licorice, candy corn, jelly beans) are still fairly energy dense, but less so than high-fat candies.

ENERGY DENSITY SPECTRUM

3.2 —————— 5.6

Candy	Serving Size	Calories	E.D. (cal/g)
Marshmallows	4 items	92	3.2
Twizzlers, cherry	2.5 oz.	242	3.4
Candy corn	1/4 cup	182	3.6
Jelly beans, large	10 pieces	104	3.7
Caramel	6 pieces	271	3.8

Candy	Serving Size	Calories	E.D. (cal/g)
Hard candy, flavored	2 pieces	47	3.9
Milky Way	2.15 oz. bar	280	4.6
Butterfinger	2.16 oz. bar	280	4.7
Snickers	2.16 oz. bar	291	4.8
Chocolate chips, semisweet	⅛ cup	102	4.8
M&M's, plain	69 pieces (1.69 oz.)	236	4.9
Almond Joy	1.7 oz. bar	246	5.0
M&M's, peanut	25 pieces (1.74 oz.)	253	5.2
Chocolate bar, milk with crisped rice	1 bar (1.5 oz.)	230	5.2
Chocolate bar, milk	1 bar (1.5 oz.)	233	5.4
Reese's Peanut Butter Cup	2 pieces (1.8 oz.)	271	5.4
Chocolate bar, milk with almonds	1 bar (1.5 oz.)	228	5.6

Part 5:

The Menu Plan

Our plan provides a base of 1,600 calories, with suggestions to provide a 2,000-calorie level. We'll also show you how to use it for different calorie levels. If you haven't done so already, please read "Creating Your Own Weight Management Program" (p. 25) and especially "How Many Calories Do You Need?" (p. 32) to get a clear idea of an appropriate calorie goal.

The 1,600 calorie plan:

400-calorie breakfast.

500-calorie lunch.

500-calorie dinner.

200 calories of *Volumetric* snacks. These can be eaten at any time of the day or evening, as two 100-calorie snacks or one 200-calorie snack. This category includes dessert.

The 2,000 calorie plan provides additional foods at lunch and dinner, and more snacks:

400-calorie breakfast.

600-calorie lunch.

600-calorie dinner.

400 calories of snacks, including dessert.

The Menu Plan can easily be modified for lower or higher calorie levels, as we'll explain in a moment. This is not a conventional diet that tells you what to eat at each meal of each day. Instead, the plan is flexible. It is modular: Each of the breakfasts contains the same number of calories, as do each of the lunches, each of the dinners, and each of the snacks. So you can interchange one lunch for another, for example. We provide you with twelve breakfasts of 400 calories, ten lunches of 500 calories, twenty-five dinners of 500 calories, and dozens of snacks under 100 or 200 calories.

These menu plans also take advantage of modular lists of

soups, vegetable side dishes, and first-course soups, which follow the menu plans. For example, rather than suggest you start lunch with a specific soup, we let you pick from any of several 100-calorie portions of soup for a first course.

Some of these menus use *Volumetric* recipes, which follow. Some include instructions for making specific dishes. Still others require no cooking at all. Wherever possible, we've given you the choice to use purchased food instead of a recipe. Many of the recipes themselves are designed to be made in advance, refrigerated or frozen, and used in single portions.

For each day, you can pick any breakfast, lunch, and dinner, and any snacks at your calorie level. You can also interchange a lunch for a dinner or vice versa. We want to give you as much freedom as possible so you can make your weight loss plan a normal part of your life. If you like three or four of the lunches, you can stick with these for weeks at a time. On the other hand, if you like variety, there are dozens of choices. It's *your* plan.

DIFFERENT CALORIE LEVELS

While we have written this plan for 1,600- and 2,000-calorie levels, it is designed to be modified for whatever calorie level you need. It's easy to add or subtract snacks, either as an appetizer or part of a meal, as a between-meal snack, or as a desert. Here's how to customize the plan:

1,400 calories. Use the 1,600-calorie plan, but drop the snacks. (We don't recommend going below 1,400 calories, because it is hard to maintain nutritional adequacy or to feel full below that level.)

1,600 calories. Use the 1,600-calorie plan.

1,800 calories. Use the 1,600 calorie plan with 400 calories of snacks.

2,000 calories. Use the 2,000 calorie plan.

2,200 calories. Main meals contain more protein and more nutrients than most snacks, so increase the portion size of breakfast and dinner. For breakfasts that call for 100 calories of fruit, eat 1½ portions of the main entrée; for those that call for fewer than 100 calories of fruit, add an extra 100 calories of fruit. Keep lunch the same. For dinner, eat 1½ servings from the main course at dinner, such as Chili Ranchero or Four-Cheese Lasagna; if the dinner menu calls for a protein food and a starchy vegetable, such as salmon and a baked potato (dinner #25, p. 172), eat 1½ portions of both. Include 300 calories of snacks.

2,400 calories. Follow the 2,200-calorie plan, but eat 2 servings at dinner. Keep snacks at 300 calories.

2,600 calories. Follow the 2,200-calorie plan, but eat 2 servings at dinner, and include 500 calories of snacks, spread throughout the day, and not all as dessert.

BEVERAGES

What about beverages? Except for coffee and tea for breakfast, and an occasional glass of juice, these menus do not include caloric beverages such as soft drinks or alcoholic beverages. We recommend water, or noncaloric drinks such as diet soda. If you want a soft drink, a glass of wine, or a beer, that's fine; consider it a snack (most 12-ounce sodas are about 150 calories), and skip a snack.

If you drink low-fat or skim milk, please continue to do so. These are excellent sources of protein and calcium. Our breakfasts, with low-fat milk or yogurt, are rich in calcium, and lunches and dinners include dairy foods, but drinking low-fat or skim milk is a good idea as well. A cup of skim or low-fat milk has around 100 calories. If you are on the 2,000-calorie plan, you can have a glass of milk with the basic 500-calorie lunch or dinner to reach your desired 600 calories. Or have a glass of milk with a 100-calorie snack to count for a 200-calorie snack.

Once you've achieved your weight loss goal, you can use this plan for maintenance at the calorie level that's appropriate for your new lower body weight. (Go back and use "How Many Calories Do You Need?" p. 32, to recalculate.) By that time, this way of eating shouldn't feel like a program for you, just the way you eat.

A few more tips:

- Eat everything at each meal. You're supposed to feel full!

- At any meal, you can eat more vegetables (except starchy ones like potatoes and corn) while only slightly increasing your calorie intake.

- To cut calories further, use skim (fat-free) milk instead of low-fat (1 percent), sugar substitutes instead of sugar, and reduced-fat or fat-free margarine.

- Use a nonstick pan to cook with little added fat.

- Add flavor without calories by using spices, herbs, garlic, vinegar, black pepper, and lemon juice.

- Because these meals aren't full of special "diet" foods, it's easy to share them with a spouse, a friend, or other family members. If others need more calories, just increase portion size.

- This is a weight loss plan for adults. Although the meals are suitable for families, including those with children, this plan is not designed for children who need to lose weight. Talk to your child's pediatrician before putting him or her on a weight-loss program.

- Don't worry about counting calories exactly, but pay attention to portion size. The proportions of foods we specify are designed to maintain the appropriate calorie levels. You don't have to measure everything perfectly for this weight loss plan to work.

Our goal is to show you a way of eating that can fill you up on fewer calories, so you can lose weight without a feeling of deprivation. Even more important, we want to show you how enjoyable this eating lifestyle can be, whether you are losing weight or preventing weight gain.

We encourage those of you who aren't planning a formal weight loss plan to try some of these menus as well as the recipes. Even if you eat a *Volumetric* dinner only once a week, you'll be learning a new way of eating. Let's start!

Menus

TWELVE BREAKFASTS OF 400 CALORIES

Whether you are on a 1,600- or 2,000-calorie plan, you should eat a filling, 400-calorie breakfast. Enjoy any of these, with any of the variations suggested, on any day of the week.

1. COLD CEREAL WITH FRUIT

Any cereal from "Breakfast Cereals of 200 Calories" (p. 177).

1 cup low-fat (1 percent) or skim milk.

100 calories of fruit from "Fruits of 100 Calories or Less" (p. 178).

1 teaspoon sugar (optional).

Coffee or tea.

2. HOT OATMEAL WITH BROWN SUGAR

1⅓ cups oatmeal, prepared with water.

1 cup low-fat (1 percent) milk.

½ grapefruit, plus ½ apple added to the oatmeal, or any 100 calories of fruit from "Fruits of 100 Calories or Less" (p. 178).

1 teaspoon ground cinnamon.

2 teaspoon brown sugar.

Coffee or tea.

3. TOASTER WAFFLES WITH FRUIT

2 fat-free or low-fat waffles.

1 cup strawberries and ¾ cup blueberries, or any 100 calories of fruit from "Fruits of 100 Calories or Less" (p. 178).

1 cup low-fat (1 percent) milk.

Coffee or tea.

4. ENGLISH MUFFIN AND FRUIT SALAD

1 English muffin.

2 teaspoons low-calorie margarine.

4 teaspoons low-sugar jam or preserves.

Citrus fruit Salad: 1 orange peeled and divided into slices, ½ grapefruit peeled and divided into slices, or any 100 calories of fruit from "Fruits of 100 Calories or Less" (p. 178).

1 cup low-fat (1 percent) milk.

Coffee or tea.

5. YOGURT AND FRUIT WITH GRANOLA

¾ cup nonfat plain yogurt.

1 medium peach, sliced, or any 100 calories of fruit from "Fruits of 100 Calories or Less" (p. 178).

2 tablespoons low-fat granola.

2 teaspoons honey.

¾ cup orange juice.

Coffee or tea.

Note: Combine the yogurt, fruit, and honey; top with the granola. The orange juice is for drinking.

6. BRAN MUFFIN AND FRUIT

1½ Double Bran, Zucchini Spice, or Blueberry-Orange Muffin (p. 248).

Any fruit from "Fruits of 100 Calories or Less" (p. 178).

1 cup low-fat (1 percent) milk.

Coffee or tea.

7. SMOOTHIE SAILING

1 serving smoothie such as Strawberry Banana (p. 246) or Pineapple Peach (p. 247).

1 English muffin, toasted, with 1 teaspoon butter or two teaspoons low-calorie soft margarine.

Coffee or tea.

8. WHOLE-WHEAT TOAST AND FRUIT

Choose any bread with about 70 calories per slice.

2 slices whole-wheat bread, toasted.

4 teaspoons low-sugar preserves.

100 calories of fruit from "Fruits of 100 Calories or Less" (p. 178).

1 cup low-fat (1 percent) milk.

Coffee or tea.

9. VEGETABLE FRITTATA

This is a nice one to serve on the weekend, when you have more time to cook.

1 serving Vegetable Frittata (p. 250).

Any 75-calorie fruit salad from "Fruits of 100 Calories or Less" (p. 178), such as ½ kiwi fruit, ¼ cup red grapes, and diced peach per serving.

1 cup low-fat (1 percent) milk.

Coffee or tea.

10. HUEVOS RANCHEROS AND FRUIT

1 serving Huevos Rancheros (p. 251).

1 cup strawberries.

1 cup low-fat (1 percent) milk.

Coffee or tea.

11. VEGETABLE OMELET WITH FRUIT

1 serving Vegetable Omelet (p. 252).

1 slice whole-wheat bread, toasted.

2 teaspoons low-sugar preserves.

1 cup diced melon.

1 cup low-fat (1 percent) milk.

Coffee or tea.

12. SCRAMBLED EGG WITH CANADIAN BACON

1 egg plus 2 egg whites (or ½ cup egg substitute) plus 2 tablespoons water, scrambled with 1 ounce Canadian bacon.

1 slice whole-wheat toast.

2 teaspoons low-sugar preserves.

1 grapefruit, sectioned or halved.

l cup low-fat (1 percent) milk.

Coffee or tea.

TEN LUNCHES OF 500 CALORIES

As with our breakfasts and dinners, you can have any of these
lunches on any day. The basic lunch menus provide 500 calories,
with suggestions for increasing the calorie count to 600.

1. SOUP AND SANDWICH

Any choice from "100-Calorie First-Course Soups"
(p. 189).

Deli sandwich: 2 slices whole-wheat bread, 6 slices deli-
thin sliced lean smoked turkey breast,* 2 pieces lettuce
(or more), 3 slices tomato, 1 tablespoon alfalfa sprouts,
1 ounce reduced-fat Cheddar cheese, 2 teaspoons mustard.

Any vegetable from "Raw Vegetables Under 30 Calories"
(p. 179), such as about 8 baby carrots.

About 60 calories of fruit: ¾ cup blueberries, or 1 cup
grapes, 1 orange, or 1¾ cups strawberries. See "Fruits of
100 Calories or Less" (p. 178).

FOR 600-CALORIE LUNCH: *Drink one cup low-fat (1 percent)
or fat-free milk, or double soup serving, or have more fruit:
1 banana; 1 pear; 1 cup cantaloupe and 1 cup honeydew melon;
1 peach, ½ cup blueberries, and ½ cup strawberries; 1 orange
and ½ grapefruit; ½ cup grapes, ½ kiwi and ½ apple (each choice
about 100 calories). Or make any choice from "100-Calorie
Snacks" (p. 173).*

*You can substitute any of the following meats: 6 slices deli-thin very lean
ham or lean roast beef. Look for turkey, ham. or roast beef with no more
than 1.5 grams of fat for 6 slices.*

2. GRILLED CHICKEN SALAD

Chicken salad: Top 3 cups romaine lettuce with ¼ cup
sliced cucumber, 4 slices green or red bell pepper, 2 tablespoons crumbled blue cheese, 1 tablespoon coarsely
chopped walnuts, and 3 ounces grilled chicken breast.

Dress with 2 tablespoons Tomato Herb Vinaigrette
(p. 214) or Creamy Cucumber Ranch Dressing (p. 212),
or low-calorie commercial salad dressing.

1 whole-wheat pita bread (6-inch).

About 40 calories of fruit, such as 1 peach, 1 plum,
½ grapefruit, or 1 cup strawberries. See "Fruits of
100 Calories or Less" (p. 178).

FOR 600-CALORIE LUNCH: *Any choice from "100-Calorie
First-Course Soups" (p. 189), or any choice from "100-Calorie
Snacks" (p. 173), or a cup low-fat (1 percent) or fat-free milk.*

3. SOUP AND VEGETARIAN BURGER

Any choice from "100-Calorie First-Course Soups"
(p. 189).

Vegetarian burger cooked without added fat (such as
oven roasting, or broiling), topped with 1 ounce part-
skim mozzarella, 1 piece romaine lettuce, 2 slices tomato,
and 1 tablespoon barbecue sauce on a whole-wheat bun.

Fruit salad (about 80 calories): ½ apple, ¼ cup grapes,
and ¼ cup blueberries; ½ cup pineapple, ½ kiwi, and
¾ cup strawberries; 1 peach, ¼ cup blueberries, and
½ cup raspberries; ½ cup honeydew, ½ cup cantaloupe,
and ⅓ cup grapes; or ½ banana and ½ orange. See
"Fruits of 100 Calories or Less" (p. 178).

FOR 600-CALORIE LUNCH: *Any choice from "100-Calorie
Snacks" (p. 173), or a cup low-fat (1 percent) or fat-free milk.*

4. SPINACH SALAD AND PITA BREAD

Spinach salad: 3 cups fresh spinach, ¼ cup sliced mushrooms, ⅓ cup garbanzo beans, ½ cup orange sections,
and 2 tablespoons feta cheese, tossed with 2 tablespoons
Citrus Vinaigrette (p. 213), or up to 4 tablespoons either
Tomato Herb Vinaigrette (p. 214) or Creamy Cucumber
Ranch Dressing (p. 212), or about 80 calories of a commercial salad dressing (check the nutrition label).

½ whole-wheat pita bread (6-inch).

About 80 calories of fruit: 1 apple, 1 cup pineapple,
1¼ cups honeydew, 2 peaches, or 2 plums. See "Fruits of
100 Calories or Less" (p. 178).

4 reduced-fat vanilla wafers.

FOR 600-CALORIE LUNCH: *Any choice from "100-Calorie
Snacks" (p. 173), or "100-Calorie First-Course Soups" (p. 189),
or a cup low-fat (1 percent) or fat-free milk.*

5. BEAN AND CHEESE BURRITO

1 Bean and Cheese Burrito (p. 234).

8 baked tortilla chips with ¼ cup salsa.

About 80 calories of fruit: 1 apple, 1 small banana,
¾ cup sweet cherries, 2 peaches, or 2 plums. See "Fruits
of 100 Calories or Less" (p. 178).

FOR 600-CALORIE LUNCH: *Any choice from "100-Calorie
Snacks" (p. 173) or "100-Calorie First-Course Soups" (p. 189),
or 1 cup low-fat (1 percent) or fat-free milk.*

6. TUNA RANCH SALAD

1 portion Tuna Ranch Salad (p. 229).

60 calories of any mix of vegetables from "Raw
Vegetables Under 30 Calories" (p. 179).

½ whole-wheat pita bread (6-inch).

About 80 calories of fruit, such as 2¼ cups strawberries,
1 apple, 1 grapefruit, 2 peaches, or 1 small banana. See
"Fruits of 100 Calories or Less" (p. 178).

FOR 600-CALORIE LUNCH: *Any choice from "100-Calorie
Snacks" (p. 173), or "100-Calorie First Course Soups" (p. 189),
or 1 cup low-fat (1 percent) or fat-free milk.*

7. BAKED POTATO WITH BROCCOLI AND CHEESE

Baked potato: Top 1 baked potato with 1 teaspoon butter (or soft tub margarine), 1 cup lightly cooked broccoli (microwave for 2–3 minutes) and ¼ cup (1 ounce) reduced-fat Cheddar cheese.

Tossed salad: Combine 2 cups lettuce, ¼ cup sliced cucumber, and ¼ cup grated carrots, dressed with 2 tablespoons Tomato Herb Vinaigrette (p. 214), Creamy Cucumber Ranch Dressing (p. 212), or about 40 calories of a commercial salad dressing.

About 40 calories of fruit: ¾ cup raspberries, 1 peach, 1 plum, or 1 cup strawberries. See "Fruits of 100 Calories or Less" (p. 178).

FOR 600-CALORIE LUNCH: *Any choice from "100-Calorie Snacks" (p. 173), or "100-Calorie First-Course Soups" (p. 189), or 1 cup low-fat (1 percent) or fat-free milk.*

8. SOUP AND CHICKEN-AND-FRUIT SALAD

Any choice from "100-Calorie First-Course Soups" (p. 189).

1 serving (1 cup) of Chicken and Fruit Salad (p. 226) on 2 slices cracked wheat bread topped with sliced tomato, lettuce, and sliced cucumber.

About 30 calories of vegetables (see "Raw Vegetables Under 30 Calories" (p. 179), such as about 8 baby carrots, or 1 stalk celery, ½ cup cucumber, and ½ cup raw broccoli.

About 40 calories of fruit: 1 plum, ½ grapefruit, ⅔ cup honeydew, or ¾ cup cantaloupe. See "Fruits of 100 Calories or Less" (p. 178).

FOR 600-CALORIE LUNCH: *Any choice from "100-Calorie Snacks" (p. 173), or 1 cup low-fat (1 percent) or fat-free milk.*

9. Taco Salad

Taco salad: In a microwave-safe bowl, stir together
½ cup of black beans, 2 tablespoons salsa, ½ teaspoon
ground cumin, and hot sauce to taste; microwave on high
approximately 40 seconds or until hot. Arrange 12 baked
tortilla chips on the bottom of a microwave-safe plate;
top with ¼ cup (1 ounce) reduced-fat Cheddar cheese;
microwave on high approximately 20 seconds or until
cheese is melted. Top the chips and cheese with the black
bean mixture, 2 cups lettuce, ½ tomato (chopped),
¼ cup salsa, and 2 tablespoons fat-free sour cream.

1 fruit-flavored sugar-free yogurt.

About 40 calories of fruit: 1 cup strawberries, ½ grapefruit, 1 peach, or ¾ cup cantaloupe. See "Fruits of 100
Calories or Less" (p. 178).

600-CALORIE LUNCH: *Any choice from "100-Calorie Snacks"
(p. 173), or "100-Calorie First-Course Soups" (p. 189), or 1 cup
low-fat (1 percent) or fat-free milk.*

10. Soup and Veggie Sandwich

Any choice from "100-Calorie First-Course Soups"
(p. 189).

Veggie sandwich: Top 2 slices whole-wheat bread with
2 ounces part-skim mozzarella cheese, 3 slices tomato,
2 pieces lettuce, 2 slices green or red pepper, 4 slices
cucumber, 1 teaspoon vinegar, ¼ teaspoon dried basil,
and ¼ teaspoon dried oregano.

About 30 calories of vegetables. See "Raw Vegetables
Under 30 Calories" (p. 179).

About 80 calories of fruit, such as 1 apple, 1 small pear,
1 small banana, or combination of ¾ cup cantaloupe and
¾ cup honeydew. See "Fruits of 100 Calories or Less"
(p. 178).

600-CALORIE LUNCH: *Any choice from "100-Calorie Snacks"
(p. 173), or 1 cup low-fat (1 percent) or fat-free milk.*

TWENTY-FIVE DINNERS OF 500 CALORIES

As with breakfasts and lunches, any of these dinner menus are fine for any night. They are entirely interchangeable. Unless otherwise noted, you should have 1 serving from any dish that calls for a recipe.

1. BURGER AND SPUDS

Great American *Volumetric* Burger (p. 217).

1 serving Creamy and Crunchy Potato Salad (p. 207), or any choice from "Vegetable Side Dishes Under 100 Calories" (p. 180), or a side salad, such as the Basic Dinner Salad with Fruit (p. 205) served with 1 tablespoon Citrus Vinaigrette (p. 213).

FOR 600-CALORIE DINNER: *Any choice from "100-Calorie First-Course Soups" (p. 189), or any choice from "Vegetable Side Dishes Under 100 Calories" (p. 180), or 1 ear corn on the cob with 1 teaspoon whipped butter.*

2. CHILI AND CITRUS

Chili Ranchero (p. 218).

Basic Dinner Salad with Fruit (p. 205) with 2 tablespoons Citrus Vinaigrette (p. 213) or commercial low-calorie salad dressing.

¾ cup tangelo segments (or segments from 1 orange if tangelo is not available).

FOR 600-CALORIE DINNER: *Add ½ cup cooked long grain rice, or a 1-ounce slice French bread (¾-inch thick) and 1 teaspoon whipped butter, or any choice from "Vegetable Side Dishes Under 100 Calories" (p. 180).*

3. LASAGNA

Four-Cheese Vegetable Lasagna (p. 231).

1 serving Fruit Soup (p. 193).

Basic Dinner Salad with Vegetables (p. 204), with
2 tablespoons Tomato Herb Vinaigrette (p. 214),
or commercial low-calorie salad dressing.

1 (1-ounce) slice French bread or baguette,
¾-inch thick.

FOR 600-CALORIE DINNER: *Add 1 cup green beans and
1 more slice French bread, or any choice from "Vegetable Side
Dishes Under 100 Calories" (p. 180)*

4. STIR-FRY WITH PORK

Stir-Fry (p. 221), made with pork. (Note: You can also
use any of the other protein sources suggested in the
recipe: beef, chicken, or tofu.)

¾ cup rice (or ½ cup cooked Oriental noodles).

Salad: Combine 2 cups torn fresh spinach, ⅓ cup drained
mandarin oranges, 1 teaspoon sliced almonds (toasted if
desired) with 1 tablespoon Citrus Vinaigrette (p. 213) or
commercial low-calorie salad dressing.

FOR 600-CALORIE DINNER: *Any choice from "100-Calorie
First-Course Soups" (p. 189), or increase the portion of the stir-fry
to 1½ servings.*

5. PASTA PRIMAVERA WITH CHICKEN

Toss Pasta Primavera (p. 235), with 3 ounces roasted
chicken breast. (If desired, serve chicken as a separate
dish.)

Fruit salad: 1 cup sliced fresh strawberries mixed with
½ cup vanilla low-fat yogurt

FOR 600-CALORIE DINNER: *Any choice from "100-Calorie
First-Course Soups" (p. 189), or add a 1-ounce slice French bread,
¾-inch thick, with 1 teaspoon whipped butter.*

6. CALYPSO NIGHT

 Gazpacho (p. 194)

 Calypso Chicken Package (p. 223)

 ½ cup cooked rice

 ½ cup honeydew melon

FOR 600-CALORIE DINNER: *Any choice from "100-Calorie First-Course Soups" (p. 189) or a 1-ounce slice French bread, ¾-inch thick, with 1 teaspoon whipped butter, or any choice from "Vegetable Side Dishes Under 100 Calories" (p. 180).*

7. FISH IN PROVENCE

 Baked Red Snapper Provencale (p. 227).

 ¾ cup cooked fettucine, tossed with 1 teaspoon olive oil.

 Sliced cucumber salad: 1 medium cucumber tossed with ½ teaspoon garlic salt (or ½ small garlic clove, minced fine) and ½ cup plain nonfat or low-fat yogurt.

FOR 600-CALORIE DINNER: *Any choice from "100-Calorie First-Course Soups" (p. 189), or any choice from "Vegetable Side Dishes Under 100 Calories" (p. 180), or a 1-ounce slice French bread, ¾-inch thick, with 1 teaspoon whipped butter*

8. PIZZA PARTY

 1½ slices *Volumetric* Pizza (p. 230), without Canadian bacon. (Note: With Canadian bacon, this dinner is 534 calories.)

 "Angel hair" cabbage-carrot slaw: Combine 1 cup shredded cabbage, ½ cup shredded carrot, 2 tablespoons fat-free or reduced-fat Italian dressing.

FOR 600-CALORIE DINNER: *Any choice from "100-Calorie First-Course Soups" (p. 189), or increase pizza slice to 2 slices.*

9. CHICKEN POT PIE

> Chicken Pot Pie (p. 224)
>
> 1 cup Waldorf Salad (p. 209)

FOR 600-CALORIE DINNER: *Any choice from "Vegetable Side Dishes Under 100 Calories" (p. 180).*

10. BACKYARD COOKOUT

> Steak and Vegetable Kabobs (p. 215).
>
> Any choice from "Vegetable Side Dishes Under 100 Calories" (p. 180).
>
> Romaine lettuce salad: Toss 1½ cups lettuce with ¼ small red onion, sliced, 2 tablespoons Caesar Salad Dressing (p. 212) or low-calorie commercial salad dressing.
>
> ½ cup watermelon, or ½ cup strawberries.

FOR 600-CALORIE DINNER: *Instead of a 100-calorie vegetable side dish, make any choice from "Vegetable Side Dishes Under 150 Calories" (p. 186), such as potato or sweet potato, and increase the fruit to 1½ cups watermelon or 1½ cups strawberries.*

11. VEGETARIAN CURRY

> Vegetable Curry Soup (p. 199), made with the vegetarian main dish variation.
>
> Spinach Salad with Mangoes: 1½ cups torn fresh spinach, sliced mango or papaya (three ½-inch slices or ½ cup cubed), 1 teaspoon sliced almonds (toast if desired), with 2 tablespoons Citrus Vinaigrette (p. 213), or commercial low-calorie dressing. (If you make the vinaigrette recipe, you may want to use pureed mango instead of orange juice for this salad.)

FOR 600-CALORIE DINNER: *Increase the couscous in the main dish soup variation to 1 cup, or add a 1-ounce slice French bread, ½-inch thick, with 1 teaspoon whipped butter.*

12. MOROCCAN GARDEN PARTY

Moroccan Garden Couscous (p. 208).

2½ ounces roasted white-meat chicken or
3 ounces broiled salmon.

Fruit Salad (p. 210), with 1 tablespoon Citrus Vinaigrette
(p. 213).

FOR 600-CALORIE DINNER: *Any choice from "100-Calorie First-Course Soups" (p. 189), or "Vegetable Side Dishes Under 100 Calories" (p. 180).*

13. CHEF'S SALAD

Chef's Salad (p. 206), tossed with 2 tablespoons
Citrus Vinaigrette (p. 213).

1 whole-wheat pita bread (6-inch) with ¼ cup Hummus
(p. 192).

¾ cup strawberries, or ½ cup diced cantaloupe
or watermelon.

FOR 600-CALORIE DINNER: *Any choice from "100-Calorie First Course Soups" (p. 189), or increase the hummus to ½ cup, or omit fruit and include any choice from "Vegetable Side Dishes Under 150 Calories" (p. 186).*

14. POULTRY AND PEANUTS

Peanut Chicken Stew (p. 225)

½ cup cooked rice

½ whole-wheat pita (6-inch), warmed

FOR 600-CALORIE DINNER: *Add 1 large apple.*

15. STEAK SOUP DINNER

Mushroom Barley Soup (p. 201), made with steak main dish variation.

Tortilla Roll-Up: Spread ¼ cup fat-free roasted-garlic cream cheese on 10-inch flour tortilla, layer ½ cup thinly sliced cucumber and 2 spinach or romaine lettuce leaves on top; roll up.

FOR 600-CALORIE DINNER: *Add a citrus fruit salad of segments from 1 orange and sections from ½ grapefruit, or any choice from "Vegetable Side Dishes Under 100 Calories" (p. 180).*

16. TURKEY SOUP DINNER

Roast Turkey Soup (p. 203).

Romaine salad: 1½ cups torn romaine lettuce and ¼ small onion, sliced, 1 ounce reduced-fat Cheddar cheese, with 2 tablespoons Creamy Cucumber Ranch Dressing (p. 212) or commercial low-calorie dressing.

1 1-ounce slice Tuscan or French bread, ¾-inch thick, with 1 teaspoon whipped butter

¾ cup frozen strawberries with 2 tablespoons frozen low-calorie whipped topping

FOR 600-CALORIE DINNER: *Increase the soup to 3 cups, or increase the bread to 2 slices with 2 teaspoons whipped butter.*

17. CHOWDER POWER

Corn Chowder (p. 200), made with the salmon main dish variation.

Tabouli: Chop finely 1 cup parsley leaves, ½ small cucumber, 1 medium tomato, 1 green onion; mix with ¼ cup soaked bulgur, 1½ teaspoons lemon juice, 1 teaspoon olive oil, and ¼ teaspoon salt. Serve on lettuce leaf.

1 apple

FOR 600-CALORIE DINNER: *Increase chowder serving to 3 cups.*

Pasta with vegetables: Top 1 cup cooked spaghetti with a quick vegetable sauté: Sauté 1 cup thinly sliced zucchini and ½ cup sliced fresh mushrooms in 1 tablespoon olive oil in a medium skillet over medium heat for 3 minutes. Stir in ½ cup canned, undrained diced tomatoes with basil, garlic, and oregano; season with ¼ teaspoon salt and pepper. Cook 3–4 minutes or until vegetables are tender, stirring frequently. Toss with the pasta and 1 tablespoon grated Parmesan cheese.

Romaine salad: Toss together 1½ cups romaine lettuce and ½ cup Category 1 vegetables (p. 107) (for example, ⅛ cup diced tomato, ⅛ cup grated carrots, ⅛ cup cucumber slices, ⅛ cup sliced red or green bell peppers), and 2 tablespoons commercial fat-free red wine vinegar salad dressing.

1 1-ounce slice Italian bread, about ¾-inch thick.

FOR 600-CALORIE DINNER: *Any choice from "100-Calorie First-Course Soups" (p. 189), or increase spaghetti to 1½ cups and increase diced tomatoes to ¾ cup.*

Grilled chicken breast: Baste one (4 ounce) skinned and boned raw chicken breast half with a mixture of 1 tablespoon lemon juice, 2 teaspoons olive oil, ½ teaspoon pepper, and ¼ teaspoon crushed dried rosemary. Grill over medium hot coals 5–6 minutes on each side (or bake, covered, at 350 degrees F. 25–30 minutes), until the chicken is no longer pink and juices run clear.

⅔ cup cooked brown rice.

1 cup broccoli florets and 1 cup sliced carrots, steamed.

1 small whole-wheat dinner roll (1 ounce).

FOR 600-CALORIE DINNER: *Any choice from "100-Calorie First-Course Soups" (p. 189), or increase the cooked brown rice to 1 cup, increase the broccoli to 1½ cups and the sliced carrots to 1¼ cups, or any choice from "Vegetable Side Dishes Under 100 calories" (p. 180).*

20. GRILLED PORK CHOP

Grilled pork chop: Baste one (4 ounce) lean, boneless pork loin with a mixture of 3 tablespoons orange juice and 1 tablespoon reduced-sodium soy sauce. Grill over medium-hot coals 20–25 minutes on each side (or bake at 350 degrees F for 35–40 minutes) or until done. Serve with ⅔ cup applesauce.

10 asparagus spears, steamed, with 1 teaspoon lemon juice and 1 teaspoon balsamic vinegar.

1 medium baked potato (about 7 ounces) with 3 tablespoons reduced-fat sour cream, salt, pepper, and, if available, chives. (Alternatives: 2 teaspoons whipped butter, 1 tablespoon reduced-calorie soft margarine, 2 tablespoons regular sour cream, or 4 tablespoons fat-free sour cream.) Or top with 4 tablespoons salsa, Worcestershire sauce, salt, pepper, and, if available, chives. Or any choice from "Vegetable Dishes Under 150 Calories" (p. 186).

FOR 600-CALORIE DINNER: *Any choice from "100-Calorie First-Course Soups" (p. 189), or increase the asparagus to 15 spears and the applesauce to 1 cup, and add 1 cup steamed carrots.*

21. STEAK FAJITA

Steak fajita: Coat a nonstick skillet with vegetable cooking spray; place over medium-high heat until hot. Add 3½ ounces lean sirloin steak strips and sauté until no longer pink. Add ½ cup thinly sliced green peppers, ½ cup thinly sliced onion, and 1 teaspoon ground cumin; sauté until the vegetables are tender. Stir in 1 tablespoon low-sodium soy sauce, 2 tablespoons commercial salsa, and hot sauce to taste; remove from heat. Layer the steak mixture, ½ cup shredded romaine or leaf lettuce, ½ cup diced tomatoes, 2 tablespoons commercial salsa, and 2 tablespoons nonfat sour cream on a 10-inch, fat-free flour tortilla; roll up.

½ cup drained, canned corn, heated.

1 cup diced cantaloupe.

FOR 600-CALORIE DINNER: *Any choice from "100-Calorie First-Course Soups" (p. 189), or add ½ cup cooked black beans, or ½ cup cooked brown or white rice, or any choice from "Vegetable Side Dishes Under 100 Calories" (p. 180).*

22. FISH FILLET DINNER

1¼ cups vegetarian vegetable soup (or any choice from "100-Calorie First-Course Soups" (p. 189).

Broiled fish: Brush both sides of a 4-ounce fillet of orange roughy, tilapia, or flounder with 1 teaspoon olive oil, 1 tablespoon lemon juice; sprinkle with ¼ teaspoon salt, ¼ teaspoon pepper, and ¼ teaspoon paprika. Broil 3–5 minutes on each side or until fish flakes with a fork.

⅔ cup cooked white rice.

Vegetable medley: Stir-fry ½ cup broccoli florets, ½ cup cauliflowerets, and ½ cup diagonally sliced carrots in 2 teaspoons olive oil in a large skillet over medium-high heat for 5 minutes or until crisp-tender; season with salt and pepper. Serve over rice. (Or make any choice from "Vegetable Side Dishes Under 100 Calories" (p. 180).

FOR 600-CALORIE DINNER: *Increase the broccoli florets in the stir-fry to 1 cup, the cauliflowerets to 1 cup, and the sliced carrots to ¾ cup; increase the rice to 1 cup.*

23. ROASTED TURKEY BREAST AND SWEET POTATO

3 ounces roasted turkey breast.

1 baked small sweet potato (¼ pound), with 1 teaspoon butter (or 2 teaspoons soft tub margarine).

1 cup cooked green beans.

¼ cup commercial whole-berry cranberry sauce.

1 slice whole grain bread (1 ounce) with 1 teaspoon butter (or soft tub margarine).

FOR 600-CALORIE DINNER: *Any choice from "100-Calorie First-Course Soups" (p. 189), or increase the cranberry sauce to ⅓ cup, the turkey to 4 ounces, and add ½ cup cooked carrots. Or add any choice from "Vegetable Side Dishes Under 100 Calories" (p. 180).*

24. EASY MEDITERRANEAN PASTA

¾ cup minestrone soup, or Quick Minestrone Soup (p. 195).

Toss ¾ cup hot cooked pasta (such as bow tie, fusilli, rotini, egg noodles, small shells, or penne) with ¾ cup thinly sliced fresh spinach leaves, ½ cup diced tomatoes, ¼ cup drained, canned garbanzo beans, 1½ tablespoons feta cheese, 1 tablespoon lemon juice, 2 teaspoons olive oil, ½ teaspoon dried basil, ½ teaspoon dried oregano, and ¼ teaspoon pepper.

1 slice Italian bread (1 ounce), about ¾-inch thick.

FOR 600-CALORIE DINNER: *Increase the cooked pasta to 1 cup, the sliced spinach to 1 cup, the diced tomato to ¾ cup, the garbanzo beans to ⅓ cup, and the feta cheese to 2 tablespoons. Or add any choice from "Vegetable Side Dishes Under 100 Calories" (p. 180).*

25. SALMON DINNER

3 ounces grilled or baked salmon.

1 medium baked potato (about 7 ounces) with 1 tablespoon reduced-fat sour cream, or 1½ tablespoons fat-free sour cream, or any choice from "Vegetable Side Dishes Under 150 Calories" (p. 186).

1 cup cooked green beans tossed with 1½ teaspoons toasted slivered almonds, or any choice from "Vegetable Side Dishes Under 100 Calories" (p. 180).

1 small whole-wheat dinner roll (1 ounce).

FOR 600-CALORIE DINNER: *Any choice from "100-Calorie First-Course Soups" (p. 189), or increase the salmon to 4 ounces and the green beans to 1¼ cups, or add a salad of 1½ cups torn romaine lettuce and ⅛ cup each of diced tomato, sliced carrots, cucumber, and green or red bell pepper tossed with 2 tablespoons commercial fat-free Italian salad dressing.*

Modular Food Lists

100-CALORIE SNACKS

1   Soup and crackers. This is a good mid-afternoon snack. Have 4 fat-free saltine crackers with any of the following canned soups, prepared with water:

¾ cup tomato soup.

¾ cup vegetarian vegetable soup.

¾ cup chicken noodle soup.

¾ cup beef noodle soup.

¾ cup minestrone soup.

Or with any of the following *Volumetrics* soups:

1 cup Light and Fresh Vegetable Soup (p. 196).

1 cup Gazpacho (p. 194).

1 cup Vegetable Curry Soup (p. 199).

2   Vegetables and dip. Choose any vegetable from Category 1 (p. 107), such as baby carrots, celery stalk, green pepper ring, or cucumber slices, and have with 2 tablespoons Creamy Cucumber Ranch Salad Dressing (p. 212), Ranch Salsa Dip (p. 192), Feta Tzatziki (p. 191), or any low-calorie commercial dressing, such as fat-free ranch dressing. Look for dressings with no more than 35 calories per tablespoon.

3   One frozen fruit juice bar (about 75 calories).

4   One cup Fruit Salad (p. 210).

5   1⅓ cups Fruit Salad Mold (p. 211).

6   3 cups plain, popped popcorn. Spray lightly with butter-flavored cooking spray and a little salt, or toss with soy sauce.

7   Slushes. Combine in a blender:

½ cup diet lemon-lime soda, ½ cup strawberries, ½ cup blueberries, ½ cup raspberries, ½ cup ice, 1 teaspoon honey or sugar (optional). Yields 2 cups.

½ banana, ½ cup strawberries, ½ cup ice, 1 teaspoon honey or sugar (optional). Yields 1½ cups.

½ cup sliced banana, ½ cup pineapple (canned in juice), 1½ cups ice, 1 teaspoon honey or sugar (optional).
Yield: 1¾ cups.

8   1 cup fat-free, sugar-free fruit-flavored yogurt.

9   ⅔ cup low-fat (1 percent) cottage cheese.

10   6 reduced-fat vanilla wafers.

11   ½ cup sherbet.

12   3½ (2½-inch) graham crackers.

13   Berries with whipped topping. Combine ¾ cup sliced strawberries, ½ cup blueberries, 1 teaspoon granulated sugar, and 1 tablespoon frozen low-calorie whipped topping.

14   ⅔ cup fat-free frozen yogurt.

15   ⅔ cup fruit-flavored gelatin dessert.

16   ½ cup sugar-free pudding prepared with reduced-fat (2 percent) milk

17   20 mini pretzels.

18   10 baked tortilla chips and ⅓ cup salsa.

1   Smoothies. Combine in a blender:

> ½ cup nonfat plain yogurt, ⅔ cup pineapple (canned in juice),
> ⅔ cup sliced banana, 1½ cups ice, 1 teaspoon honey or sugar
> (optional). Yield: 2½ cups.

> ½ cup fat-free strawberry yogurt, ¼ cup raspberries, ½ cup
> strawberries, ½ cup blueberries, and ¾ cup ice. Yield: 2 cups.

> ¾ cup fat-free, sugar-free yogurt, ¾ cup strawberries, ½ cup
> bananas, 1 cup ice. Yield: 2 cups.

2   Cereal and milk. This makes an easy, nutritious snack. Give
yourself a smaller portion for a snack than you would for a breakfast. Our cereals list (p. 178) with 1 cup milk provide about
300 calories, so you'll want to have only about two-thirds of
that. Example: ⅔ cup Raisin Bran or ¾ cup Multi-Bran Chex
with ½ cup low-fat (1 percent) milk. Other suggestions:

> For about 200 calories, have 1 cup Cheerios, 1 cup Crispix,
> 1 cup Rice Krispies, or 1 cup Wheaties with ⅔ cup blueberries,
> or 1 cup strawberries and ½ cup fat-free milk. Note: 1 tea-
> spoon sugar adds 15 calories.

3   Baked apple with low-fat ice cream and low-fat granola. Core a
medium apple, add ½ teaspoon lemon juice, place in a microwave-
safe dish, and cook for 2 minutes on high; serve with ½ teaspoon
ground cinnamon, ⅓ cup low-fat vanilla ice cream, and 1 tablespoon low-fat granola.

4   Vanilla frozen yogurt with fresh fruit. Have ½ cup nonfat
vanilla frozen yogurt with ⅔ cup fresh sliced peaches or ½ cup fresh
strawberries, or any fruit of less than 50 calories. See "Fruits of
100 Calories or Less" (p. 178)

5   Yogurt, granola, honey, and fruit. Combine 6 ounces fat-free
plain yogurt, 2 teaspoons honey, 1 tablespoon low-fat granola, and
any of the following fruits: ¾ cup sliced strawberries, ½ cup blue-

berries, ½ cup diced pineapple, or any fruit of less than 50 calories. See "Fruits of 100 Calories or Less" (p.178). Top yogurt with fruit, then add honey and granola.

6   Angel food cake with fruit and whipped topping. Top 1 slice (1/12 of a 10-inch cake) with 1 cup strawberries, ⅔ cup blueberries, or ¾ cup raspberries plus 2 tablespoons frozen low-calorie whipped topping.

7   Fruit smoothies and slushes. Combine these ingredients in a blender (for a thicker drink, freeze fruit first and use slightly thawed):

> Orange Banana Slush: ⅔ cup orange sherbet, ½ cup diet lemon-lime soda or seltzer, ½ cup sliced banana and ⅔ cup ice.

> Pineapple Banana Smoothie: ½ cup nonfat plain yogurt, ⅔ cup pineapple, ⅔ cup sliced banana, and ¾ cup ice.

> Three Berry Smoothie: ½ cup 99 percent fat-free fruit-flavored yogurt, ½ cup strawberries, ½ cup blueberries, ¼ cup raspberries, and ¾ cup ice.

> Strawberry Banana Smoothie: ¾ cup nonfat fruit-flavored yogurt with aspartame, ¾ cup strawberries, ½ cup sliced banana, and 1 cup ice.

8   Peaches and cottage cheese. Combine 1 cup peaches in light syrup with ½ cup low-fat (1 percent) cottage cheese.

9   Ice cream, bananas, and chocolate syrup. Combine ½ cup low-fat vanilla ice cream, ½ sliced banana, and 1 tablespoon chocolate syrup.

10   Black beans and cheese. Mix ¾ cup black beans, drained, with 3 tablespoons salsa, cover with microwave-safe plastic wrap, and heat in microwave on high for 1 minute; top with 1 teaspoon reduced-fat Cheddar cheese and heat another 30 seconds.

11 Veggie pita. Any vegetable from Category 1 (p. 107) with ¼ cup Hummus (p. 192) or commercial low-fat hummus with 1 teaspoon lemon juice on ½ whole-wheat pita bread (6-inch). Here's a suggested mix: 3 slices tomato, 2 green pepper rings, 1 leaf lettuce, ⅛ cup sliced cucumber, 1 tablespoon alfalfa sprouts. Add salt, pepper, and herbs such as oregano or fresh basil to taste.

12 Chips and bean dip. To make 4 servings: Combine ¾ cup fat-free refried beans with ½ cup salsa, spread on bottom of a serving platter; top with ¼ cup fat-free sour cream, ¼ cup reduced-fat Cheddar cheese, 1 cup shredded romaine lettuce, and 1 cup diced tomato. Sprinkle with chili powder. Serve with 32 large baked tortilla chips. If you like a hotter dish, add hot sauce and green chilies to bean mixture. Or have a ½-cup serving of Layered Black Bean Dip (p. 190) with 7 medium low-fat baked tortilla chips.

13 8 ounces Fruit-Flavored Italian Ice (140 calories).

14 Baked potato. 1 medium, hot baked potato, (about 7 ounces) topped with 2 tablespoons fat-free sour cream, salt and pepper to taste.

15 Volumetric desserts. One serving of any of the following desserts: Red, White and Blue Trifle (p. 237), Fudge Cake Brownies (p. 243), Brownie Sundae Soufflés (p. 238), Baked Pumpkin Custard (p. 245).

BREAKFAST CEREALS OF 200 CALORIES

Here are some choices for breakfast number 1 (p. 154). One cup of low-fat (1 percent) milk adds 100 calories; skim milk, 86 calories. The following cereals are low in energy density and big in volume, so you get a good portion, and are low in sugar and rich in fiber. If you want, add a teaspoon of sugar, which adds 15 calories. Top with fruit, and you'll still be under 400 calories for breakfast. (If you want to eat a breakfast cereal not on this list, look for one that gives you close to a cup or more for 200 calories and has at least 5 grams of fiber.)

Cereal	Serving Size	Fiber (in grams)
Kellogg's All-Bran	1¼ cups	25
Post Raisin Bran	1 cup	9
Post Bran Flakes	1¼ cups	9
Kellogg's Bran Flakes	2 cups	5
General Mills Multi-bran Chex	1 cup	7
Quaker Shredded Wheat	3 biscuits	7
Nabisco Shredded Wheat, original	2½ biscuit	6
General Mills Wheaties	2 cups	6
General Mills Cheerios	1¾ cups	5
General Mills Wheat Chex	¾ cup	5
Oatmeal, prepared with water	1⅓ cups	5

FRUITS OF 100 CALORIES OR LESS

Fresh fruit is a great *Volumetric* treat any time of the day or night.

For breakfast, top your cereal with any of the fruits below for about 100 calories (or less). You can also combine these fruits into a fruit salad; for example, ½ cup strawberries, ¼ cup blueberries, and ½ banana is 100 calories. So is 1 orange and ½ grapefruit.

Fruit is also an excellent addition to lunch or dinner, or as a snack.

Typical Serving	Calories
1 banana, medium	110
1 pear	100
1 apple	80
1 cup blueberries	80
1 cup pineapple	80
1 grapefruit, medium	70
1 orange, medium	60
1 cup grapes	60
1 cup honeydew	60
1 cup cantaloupe	60
1 kiwi fruit	50
1 peach	40
1 cup raspberries	40
1 plum	40
1 cup strawberries	40

RAW VEGETABLES UNDER 30 CALORIES

Use this chart to select raw vegetables to add to lunch or dinner, or to snack on. All data are for raw vegetables. For example, 1 stalk celery, ½ tomato, and ½ cup cauliflower is 30 calories; so is ¼ cup bell peppers, ½ cup broccoli, and ½ cup cucumber.

Food	Calories
Cucumber, sliced, ½ cup	10
Lettuce, shredded, 1 cup	10
Celery, 1 stalk	10
Tomato, 1 medium	30
Spinach, 1 cup	10
Cabbage, 1 cup	20
Cauliflower, ½ cup	10
Mushrooms, ½ cup	10
Peppers, green or red bell peppers, ½ cup	20
Broccoli, ½ cup	10
Alfalfa sprouts, ¼ cup	5
Onions, ¼ cup	20
Carrots, ½ cup or 8 baby carrots	30

COOKED VEGETABLE CALORIES

Most vegetables are very low in energy density. Starchy vegetables, such as lima beans, corn, sweet potatoes, and potatoes, are somewhat higher. (For cooking suggestions, see pp. 180–188).

Food	Calories
Eggplant, boiled, drained, ½ cup	10
Cauliflower, boiled, ½ cup	10
Cabbage, green, ½ cup shredded, boiled, drained	20
Summer squash (yellow squash/zucchini), boiled, ½ cup	20
Spinach, ½ cup, boiled, drained	20
Asparagus, boiled, drained, ½ cup	20
Broccoli, boiled, ½ cup	20
Green beans, steamed, ½ cup	20

Carrots, boiled, drained, ½ cup	40
Green peas, frozen, boiled, ½ cup	60
Corn, canned, boiled, ½ cup	70
Sweet potato, baked, 1 medium (4 ounces)	100
Potato, baked with skin, ½ medium (4 ounces)	110

VEGETABLE SIDE DISHES UNDER 100 CALORIES

Most vegetables are so low in calories that if you cook them with little or no added fat, you can eat a large amount for under 100 calories. Each of these suggestions makes 1 large serving.

ASPARAGUS

Amount: 3–4 spears, about 4 ounces (cut up and trimmed, about 1¼–1½ cups).

Prep: Cut off the tough ends of asparagus spears and trim spears. Using a small sharp paring knife, insert the knife under the thicker skin at the base and work it toward the tip, making cut shallower as the skin becomes thinner. Taper off peeling about 2–3 inches from the tip end.

Roasted asparagus. Preheat the oven to 450 degrees F. Cut the spears into 1½-inch lengths, or leave whole. Toss with 1 teaspoon extra-virgin olive oil and ¼ teaspoon salt, and place on a baking sheet. Bake for 10 minutes or until just tender.

Sautéed asparagus. Cut the spears into 1½-inch lengths. Coat a nonstick skillet with olive oil–flavored cooking spray, and place it over medium-high heat. Add the asparagus and 3 tablespoons minced green onion, sprinkle with ¼ teaspoon salt, and sauté 30 seconds. Add ¼ cup water; cover and steam 3–5 minutes or until the asparagus is just tender. Uncover and increase the heat; boil to evaporate the liquid. Stir in ½ teaspoon dark sesame oil or olive oil, and remove from heat.

Microwave asparagus. Arrange whole or cut up spears in a glass dish just large enough to hold them. Add 2 tablespoons water and cover tightly. Microwave on high for 2–4 minutes or until tender, rearranging spears or stirring once. Drain and toss with 1 teaspoon lemon juice, ½ teaspoon olive oil, ¼ teaspoon salt, and freshly ground pepper to taste.

BROCCOLI

Amount: 1 stalk of broccoli, about 6 ounces.

Prep: Wash, cut off the tough end of the stalk. Trim the tough outer skin of the stalk with a small sharp knife. Slice off the stalk from florets, and slice it thinly. Separate the larger florets into a smaller pieces.

Steamed broccoli. Bring 1 inch of water to a boil in a steamer or large saucepan. Fill the steamer basket or colander with broccoli, placing stalk pieces on the bottom, and place over water. Cover and steam 8–15 minutes or until tender. Toss with 1 teaspoon low-sodium soy sauce, ½ teaspoon sesame oil, and ½ teaspoon toasted sesame seeds.

Blanched broccoli. Cook the broccoli in boiling salted water 4–5 minutes or until a sharp knife easily pierces stalk pieces and broccoli is crisp-tender. Drain and toss with 2 teaspoons lemon juice, 1 teaspoon melted butter (or soft tub margarine), and, if desired, ¼ teaspoon crushed red pepper.

Microwave broccoli. Combine broccoli and ¼ cup water in a glass bowl, and cover tightly with heavy-duty plastic wrap. Microwave on high for 2–3 minutes or until crisp-tender; let stand, covered, 1 minute. Drain broccoli; toss with ¼ teaspoon salt. Drizzle with 2 teaspoons commercial reduced-calorie ranch salad dressing.

CABBAGE

Amount: About 2½–3 cups sliced cabbage, which makes about 1 cup cooked.

Prep: Remove any tough, discolored outer leaves. Cut out the core and slice thinly.

Microwave Greek-style cabbage. Combine 2½ cups sliced cabbage, ¼ cup finely chopped green onion, 2 tablespoons chicken broth, 1 teaspoon olive oil, ½ teaspoon salt, and ½ teaspoon dried oregano in a glass bowl; cover and microwave on high for 8–12 minutes or until the cabbage is tender, stirring once. Uncover, stir in 1 teaspoon lemon juice.

Stir-fried cabbage. Heat 1 teaspoon olive oil in a large nonstick skillet over medium heat. Add 1 teaspoon minced garlic and ½ teaspoon minced fresh ginger, and stir-fry 30 seconds. Add 3 cups sliced cabbage (cut paper thin, or use commercial, packaged angel-hair sliced cabbage), and stir-fry 4–5 minutes or until wilted and beginning to brown. Stir in 2 teaspoons reduced-sodium soy sauce, ½ teaspoon sesame oil, and, if desired, ½ teaspoon toasted sesame seeds.

Italian braised cabbage. Combine 2½ cups sliced cabbage, ½ cup canned Italian-style stewed tomatoes (undrained), ¼ cup chicken broth or water, and ¼ teaspoon salt in a small saucepan. Cover and cook over medium heat until cabbage is tender.

CARROTS

Amount: 1 cup sliced or chopped, about 4 ounces peeled and trimmed.

Prep: Cut off the tip and root ends of carrots; peel with vegetable peeler.

Sautéed carrots. Cut the carrots into 2-inch x ¼-inch julienne strips. Heat 1 teaspoon olive oil in a nonstick skillet over medium heat; add the carrots, ¼ teaspoon salt, and ½ teaspoon sugar, and toss to coat. Add 2 tablespoons orange juice; cover, reduce heat to low, and simmer 5 minutes or until carrots are just tender.

Stove-top carrots. Cook the sliced carrots, covered, in a small amount of boiling water for 3–5 minutes or until just tender. Drain well. Toss with a mixture of 2 tablespoons orange juice, 2 teaspoons honey, a dash of ground ginger, and, if desired, 1 teaspoon minced fresh parsley.

Microwave carrots with cranberries and apples. In a 1-quart glass bowl or baking dish, mix together 1½ cups grated carrots, ½ cored grated apple, ¼ cup frozen or fresh cranberries, 1 tablespoon water, 1 tablespoon light brown sugar, and ⅛ teaspoon salt. Cover and microwave on high 5–6 minutes, or until the carrots are just tender. Let stand, covered, 2 minutes.

CAULIFLOWER

Amount: 1 cup cauliflowerets, about 4 ounces.

Prep: Remove the leaves and trim off the thick bottom end. Hollow out the core, and break into flowerets. Trim the flowerets with a paring knife, cutting off the ends and peeling off tough stem skin if necessary. Cut the larger flowerets into ½-inch diameter pieces.

Steamed cauliflower with bread crumbs. Bring 1 inch of water to a boil in a steamer or saucepan. Place the cauliflower flowerets in a steamer basket or colander over boiling water, cover and steam 3–4 minutes or until just tender. Remove the cauliflower from the steamer and toss with a mixture of 2 tablespoons oven-toasted fresh bread crumbs, 1 teaspoon olive oil, 1 teaspoon Dijon mustard, and ½ teaspoon drained capers.

Mashed cauliflower. Cook the cauliflowerets in boiling water 3–6 minutes or until very tender. Drain; puree in a food processor with 1 tablespoon reduced-fat sour cream, ¼ teaspoon salt, and ¼ teaspoon freshly ground pepper. Reheat in a saucepan.

Microwave cauliflower. Combine ¼ cup undrained pasta-style canned chunky tomatoes and ¾ cup cauliflowerets in a small microwave-safe dish. Cover with heavy-duty plastic wrap and microwave on high 3–5 minutes or until the cauliflower is just tender, stirring once.

EGGPLANT

Amount: ½ pound per serving

Prep: Cut off the stem end of an eggplant.

Broiled eggplant slices. Cut the eggplant into ½-inch-thick slices. Coat both sides of the slices with olive oil–flavored cooking spray; place on a broiler pan rack. Sprinkle both sides of the slices with ½ teaspoon salt. Broil 5 inches from the heat source until the top is browned. Turn; coat again with cooking spray and sprinkle with mixture of 2 tablespoons minced fresh herbs and 1 teaspoon finely minced garlic. Broil until golden.

Baked eggplant slices. Preheat the oven to 425 degrees F. Cut eggplant into ¾-inch slices. Coat both sides of the slices with olive oil–flavored cooking spray; sprinkle both sides of slices with ½ teaspoon salt and arrange in a baking pan in a single layer. Bake for 5–10 minutes or until just tender. Remove from oven and top with mixture of ¼ cup diced plum tomatoes, 2 tablespoons minced green onion, 2 sliced pitted ripe olives; bake 3–5 additional minutes or until eggplant is tender.

Grilled eggplant slices. Cut the eggplant into ¾-inch-thick slices. Brush each slice with a mixture of 1 tablespoon low-sodium soy sauce, 1 teaspoon balsamic vinegar, 1 teaspoon dark sesame oil, and ¼ teaspoon garlic powder. Grill 3–5 minutes on each side or until browned and tender.

GREEN BEANS

Amount: 4 ounces.

Prep: Wash the beans and snap off the stem ends of the beans; break or cut into 2-inch lengths.

Steamed beans. Bring 1 inch of water to a boil in a steamer or saucepan. Place the beans, mixed with ¼ teaspoon dried tarragon, in a steamer basket or colander over boiling water; cover and steam 5 minutes or until just tender. Remove from steamer; toss with 1 teaspoon lemon juice, 1 teaspoon butter or soft tub margarine, ¼ teaspoon salt, and ¼ teaspoon freshly ground pepper.

Blanched beans Nicoise. Bring 1 quart water and 1½ teaspoons salt to a boil in a saucepan; add the beans. Boil 4–5 minutes or until the beans are crisp tender. Drain and toss with ¼ cup diced tomatoes, 2 tablespoons minced onion, 1 teaspoon balsamic vinegar, and ½ teaspoon olive oil.

Microwave beans. Combine the beans and ¼ cup water in a 1-quart glass dish, cover tightly with heavy-duty plastic wrap, and microwave on high 4–6 minutes or until crisp-tender, stirring once. Drain; toss with ½ teaspoon butter or soft tub margarine and 1 teaspoon toasted sliced almonds or grated Parmesan cheese.

SPINACH

Amount: 12 ounces.
Prep: Remove tough stems; wash and drain in a colander.

Steamed spinach. Boil 1 inch of water in a steamer or saucepan, and place the spinach in steamer basket or colander. Place in a steamer or saucepan and cover tightly. Cook 5 minutes. Remove from the pot; transfer to a bowl and stir in 1 teaspoon extra-virgin olive oil, 1 teaspoon lemon juice, ¼ teaspoon salt, and ¼ teaspoon freshly ground pepper.

Stir-fried Oriental spinach. Cut the spinach into wide strips. Heat 1 teaspoon canola oil in a nonstick skillet over medium-high heat; sauté 2 teaspoons grated gingerroot and 1 teaspoon minced garlic 30 seconds. Add the spinach; stir-fry 3 minutes. Reduce heat to medium; stir in 2 teaspoons reduced-sodium soy sauce and 1 teaspoon rice wine vinegar or dry sherry. Cover and cook 1–2 minutes.

Spicy microwave spinach. Place the spinach, with water clinging to leaves, in a 2-quart glass dish or bowl; cover with heavy-duty plastic wrap and microwave on high for 5–8 minutes, stirring once. Uncover and stir in 2 teaspoons butter or soft tub margarine, ¼ teaspoon salt, and hot pepper vinegar or hot sauce to taste.

SUMMER SQUASH (YELLOW SQUASH, ZUCCHINI)

Amount: 1 cup slices or cubes, about 4 ounces.
Prep: Cut off the stem ends.

Sautéed squash. Cut the squash into ½- to ¾-inch cubes. Heat 1 teaspoon olive oil in a nonstick skillet over medium heat, add the squash, and sauté 5–6 minutes. Stir in ⅓ cup canned chili-style chunky tomatoes; heat thoroughly.

Roasted squash. Preheat the oven to 450 degrees F. Cut the squash into cubes, toss with 1 teaspoon olive oil, ½ teaspoon dried oregano, ½ teaspoon salt, and ¼ teaspoon pepper, and arrange on a jellyroll pan coated with olive oil–flavored cooking spray. Bake for 10–15 minutes or until the squash is tender. Toss with 2 tablespoons thinly sliced roasted red peppers.

Grilled or broiled squash. Cut the squash lengthwise into ½-inch-thick slices, and baste with 1 tablespoon commercial fat-free red wine vinegar salad dressing. Grill over medium coals 3 minutes on each side, basting with 1 tablespoon additional salad dressing. Or place on a broiler pan rack and broil 4 inches from the heat source 2–3 minutes on each side, or until lightly browned and tender.

VEGETABLE SIDE DISHES UNDER 150 CALORIES

Starchy vegetables like green peas, corn, potatoes, and sweet potatoes are more energy dense than the nonstarchy vegetables in the list above. So these side dishes contain more calories per portion, but are still under 150 calories.

CORN

Amount: 2 medium ears of corn, ¾ cups fresh corn kernels, or ¾ cups drained, frozen, or canned corn.

Prep: Remove husks and silk; cut corn from cobs using a sharp knife.

Creamed corn. Blanch ¾ cups fresh corn kernels in boiling water 3 minutes; drain well. Do not blanch frozen or canned corn. Heat a nonstick skillet coated with vegetable cooking spray over medium-low heat; add ⅓ cup minced onion, and sauté 5 minutes. Whisk together 1 teaspoon all-purpose flour, ¼ cup evaporated fat-free milk, ¼ teaspoon salt, and ¼ teaspoon pepper; stir into corn.

Corn sauté. Heat 1 teaspoon canola oil in a nonstick skillet over medium-high heat. Add 2 tablespoons chopped green pepper, 2 tablespoons chopped onion, and ¼ teaspoon ground cumin; sauté 1 minute. Add ¾ cup corn kernels and ⅛ teaspoon salt; sauté 3–5 minutes or until corn is hot and just tender (if fresh).

Microwave corn. In a microwave-safe bowl, mix together ¾ cup corn kernels, 2 tablespoons diced celery or green pepper, 1 tablespoon diced canned pimiento (drained), and 1 teaspoon butter (or soft tub margarine). Cover tightly and microwave on high 2–3 minutes or until hot and the corn is tender (if using fresh). Uncover and stir in ⅛ teaspoon salt and pepper to taste.

GREEN PEAS

> **Amount:** ¾ cup frozen peas.
> **Prep:** Thaw.

Sautéed peas with cucumbers. Heat 1 teaspoon olive oil in a nonstick skillet over medium-high heat. Add ¾ cup peas and ¼ cup sliced cucumber (cut slices into half-moon shapes), and sauté 5 minutes. Stir in ½ teaspoon dried dillweed and ¼ teaspoon salt.

Simmered mint-flavored peas. Combine ¾ cup frozen tiny tender peas, thawed with 2 tablespoons chicken broth or water, 2 teaspoons mint jelly (optional), 1 teaspoon olive oil, and 1 teaspoon minced green onion tops, chives, or mint in a small saucepan; cook over medium heat 5–10 minutes or until peas are just tender.

Microwaved peas. Combine ¾ cup peas, ¼ cup diced red bell pepper, and 2 tablespoons water in a glass bowl; cover and microwave on high 2 minutes or until tender. Drain and toss with 1 tablespoon minced basil and ¼ teaspoon salt.

POTATO

> **Amount:** ½ medium-size baking potato, about 4 ounces, or 1 red potato (4 ounces).
> **Prep:** Scrub potato under running water.

Quick country mashed potatoes. Dice the potato and combine it with ¼ cup chopped onion, 3 tablespoons skim milk or water, ¼ teaspoon salt, and pepper in a glass bowl; cover tightly with plastic wrap. Microwave on high for 5–7 minutes or until potatoes are tender. Let stand, covered, 2 minutes. Uncover and mash with a potato masher.

Mediterranean-style baked potato chunks. Preheat the oven to 450 degrees F. Cut the potato into 1½-inch pieces, and toss with 1 teaspoon olive oil, 1 teaspoon lemon juice, ¼ teaspoon dried oregano, ¼ teaspoon salt, and pepper in a baking pan. Bake for 30 minutes or until crispy and tender, stirring once.

Seasoned oven-baked fries. Preheat the oven to 450 degrees F. Cut the potato into long, ½-inch strips, and coat with butter-flavor vegetable cooking spray on a baking sheet. Toss with ½ teaspoon seasoned salt, and spread in a single layer; coat again with cooking spray. Bake for 20 minutes, turning twice.

SWEET POTATO

Amount: 1 small sweet potato, about ¼ pound.
Prep: See recipe suggestions.

Boiled mashed sweet potatoes. Scrub the sweet potato, place it in a pot, and cover with water. Bring to a boil and cook for 25–35 minutes or until tender when pierced with a knife. Drain and peel; mash with 1 teaspoon butter, 1 teaspoon frozen orange juice concentrate, and ¼ teaspoon salt.

Baked mashed sweet potatoes. Preheat the oven to 400 degrees F. Scrub the sweet potato; pierce it several times with a fork. Bake until the sweet potato is soft when pinched, about 40–45 minutes. Cut in half lengthwise, and mash the pulp with 1 teaspoon honey, 1 teaspoon butter (or soft tub margarine), ¼ teaspoon salt, and ¼ teaspoon ground pumpkin pie spice.

Microwave maple-flavored sweet potatoes. Boil the sweet potato as directed above. Peel and cut it into ½-inch-thick slices. Arrange in a shallow, 1½-cup, microwave-proof serving dish in concentric circles, overlapping slightly. Stir together 1 tablespoon reduced-calorie pancake syrup, 2 tablespoon orange juice, and a pinch of ground cinnamon; drizzle over sweet potatoes. Cover and microwave on high for 1 minute or until hot.

100-CALORIE FIRST-COURSE SOUPS

A broth-based soup makes an excellent first course for lunch or dinner. Choose from any of the following 100 calorie first-course soups:

1½ cups Vegetable Curry Soup (p. 199).

1½ cups Gazpacho (p. 194).

1¼ cups Light and Fresh Vegetable Soup (p. 196).

1 cup Cream of Broccoli Soup (p. 197).

1 cup Roast Turkey Soup (p. 203).

You can also choose any commercial soup, as long as the calories are under 100 per serving and the serving is at least 1 full cup. Any of the following, prepared with water, are excellent choices:

1¼ cups vegetarian vegetable soup.

1¼ cups tomato soup.

1¼ cups minestrone soup.

1¼ cups vegetable beef soup.

1¼ cups chicken noodle soup.

Recipes

Layered Black Bean Dip

Serve ½ cup of this dip with raw vegetables and you can have a filling snack for under 150 calories.

1 (15-ounce) can black beans, rinsed and drained

3 tablespoons lemon juice

1 teaspoon ground cumin

1 teaspoon chili powder

¼ teaspoon salt

½ cup finely chopped water chestnuts

¼ cup chopped green onion

½ cup finely chopped red or green bell pepper

¾ cup fat-free sour cream

½ cup (2 ounces) shredded part-skim mozzarella cheese

½ cup finely chopped tomato

¼ cup finely diced cucumber

¼ cup chopped cilantro or parsley

Mash beans in a medium bowl (a potato masher works well.) Stir in the lemon juice, cumin, chili powder, salt, water chestnuts, green onion, and peppers. Spread in a shallow serving dish, cover, and refrigerate at least 2 hours.

Just before serving, spread the sour cream on the bean mixture, and top with layers of cheese, tomato, cucumber, and cilantro.

Yield: 8 servings of ½ cup each.

Nutritional Information Per Serving. Calories: 110. Energy Density: 1.0. Carbohydrate: 18 g. Fat: 1 g. Protein: 7 g. Fiber: 4 g. Sodium: 128 mg.

Feta Tzatziki

This is a lower-fat version of the classic Greek cucumber dip. Serve it with raw vegetables such as carrot sticks, cut-up celery stalks, broccoli florets, summer squash slices, or bell pepper slices. It's also good with pita bread, either very fresh and soft, or cut into small triangles and crisped in a 350 degree F. oven for 10 minutes.

- ½ large seedless European cucumber
  (or 1 standard cucumber, seeded)
- 1 clove garlic, minced
- ¼ teaspoon salt
- ½ cup (2 ounces) finely crumbled feta cheese
- 1½ cups fat-free plain yogurt
- 1 tablespoon minced fresh (or 1 teaspoon dried) dill
- 2 teaspoons white wine vinegar
- 1 teaspoon extra virgin olive oil

Wash and dry the cucumber, cut off the ends, and grate it on the large holes of a cheese grater; drain on paper towels for 1 minute. Mix the grated cucumber with the garlic and salt in a medium bowl.

Crumble the feta cheese evenly over the cucumber mixture, and stir well to blend. Stir in the yogurt, dill, vinegar, and olive oil. Cover and refrigerate at least 1 hour to blend the flavors.

Yield: 9 servings of ¼ cup each.

Nutritional Information Per Serving. Calories: 50. Energy Density: 0.7. Carbohydrate: 4 g. Fat: 2 g. Protein: 4 g. Fiber: 0 g. Sodium: 193 mg.

Hummus

As with the Feta Tzatziki (p. 191), this is good with either raw cut-up vegetables or pita bread wedges.

    ¾ cup plain fat-free yogurt
    2 cloves garlic, minced
    1 (15-ounce) can chickpeas (garbanzo beans), drained
    3 tablespoons sesame seeds, toasted
    1 tablespoon lemon juice
    1 teaspoon dark sesame oil
    ½ teaspoon salt
    ¾ teaspoon ground cumin
    ¼ teaspoon ground red pepper

Combine all the ingredients in a blender container, cover, and process until smooth, scraping the sides as necessary. Transfer to a bowl, cover, and refrigerate at least 2 hours, and up to 3 days.

Yield: 7 servings of ¼ cup each.

Nutritional Information Per Serving. Calories: 100. Energy Density: 1.5. Carbohydrate: 13 g. Fat: 4 g. Protein: 5 g. Fiber: 3 g. Sodium: 186 mg.

Ranch Salsa Dip

Serve this with baked tortilla chips or cut raw veggies.

    1 (16-ounce) carton fat-free sour cream
    1 (½-ounce) envelope ranch-style dressing mix
    ¼ cup minced cilantro
    1 cup commercial chunky salsa

Stir together the first three ingredients in a medium bowl. Stir in the salsa. Cover and refrigerate at least 2 hours, and up to 2 days.

Yield: 8 servings of ¼ cup each.

Nutritional Information Per Serving. Calories: 70. Energy Density: 1.0. Carbohydrate: 13 g. Fat: 0 g. Protein: 4 g. Fiber: 0 g. Sodium: 237 mg.

Fresh Fruit Soup

When the weather is warm, cool fruit refreshes. Try this soup as a first course, or dessert.

3 cups diced cantaloupe or honeydew melon

½ cup peach or apricot nectar

½ cup vanilla fat-free yogurt

1 tablespoon honey

2 teaspoons fresh lime juice

½ teaspoon vanilla extract

1 cup diced, peeled and pitted peaches or plums

1 cup fresh blueberries

1 cup quartered strawberries or fresh raspberries

Process the first six ingredients in a blender until smooth. Combine the mixture with the diced peaches, blueberries, and strawberries in a bowl. Cover and refrigerate at least 2 hours.

Yield: 5 servings of 1 cup each.

Note: If peaches, plums, and berries aren't in season, omit them. Add 1 (10-ounce) package frozen raspberries or strawberries and press through a sieve, discarding solids. Stir in 2 tablespoons sugar until dissolved. Spoon 1½ tablespoons of the puree into each cup of soup and swirl with the tip of a knife.

Nutritional Information Per Serving. Calories: 135. Energy Density: 0.5. Carbohydrate: 33 g. Fat: 1 g. Protein: 3 g. Fiber: 4 g. Sodium: 26 mg. Good Source: Vitamin C.

Gazpacho

1 (28-ounce) can crushed tomatoes, undrained

2 cups vegetable juice cocktail

2½ tablespoons red wine vinegar

1 tablespoon olive oil

½ teaspoon hot sauce, or more to taste

1¾ cups finely diced cucumber (about 1 large)

1 cup finely diced green or yellow bell pepper

⅓ cup minced cilantro or parsley

¼ cup minced green onions

1 or 2 cloves garlic, finely minced

Garnish: lemon wedges, cilantro or parsley sprigs (optional)

Combine the first five ingredients in a large pitcher. Stir in the cucumber, bell pepper, minced cilantro, green onion, and garlic. Cover and refrigerate at least 3 hours and up to 3 days.

Serve in large goblets. Add desired garnishes.

Yield: 4 servings of 1¾ cups each.

Nutritional Information Per Serving. Calories: 120. Energy Density: 0.3.
Carbohydrate: 21 g. Fat: 4 g. Protein: 3 g. Fiber: 4 g. Sodium: 787 mg.
Good Source: Vitamin C.

Quick Minestrone

1 tablespoon olive oil

2 cups chopped carrots

1 cup chopped onion

1 cup chopped celery

3 cloves garlic, chopped

1 (28-ounce) can crushed tomatoes, undrained

1 cup canned low-fat or fat-free chicken broth

1 cup water

1 teaspoon dried Italian seasoning

¼ teaspoon salt

2 cups packed sliced fresh spinach

1 (15-ounce) can small white (navy) beans, rinsed and drained

⅔ cup cooked small rice-shaped pasta (orzo)

Heat the olive oil in a large, heavy saucepan over medium heat. Add the carrots, onion, celery and garlic; sauté 10 minutes or until the vegetables are crisp-tender.

Stir in the tomatoes, broth, water, Italian seasoning, and salt, and bring to a boil. Cover, reduce heat, and simmer 20 minutes or until carrots are tender. Add the spinach, cover, and simmer for 5 minutes. Stir in the beans and pasta, simmer 1 minute or until hot.

Yield: 8 servings of 1 cup each.

Nutritional Information Per Serving. Calories: 130. Energy Density: 0.5. Carbohydrate: 24 g. Fat: 2 g. Protein: 6 g. Fiber: 5 g. Sodium: 414 mg. Good Source: Fiber, Vitamin A.

Light and Fresh Vegetable Soup

See below for ethnic main dish variations.

> 2 teaspoons olive oil
>
> 4 cloves garlic, minced
>
> 5 cups canned low-fat or fat-free chicken broth
>
> 2 sprigs thyme
>
> 1¾ cups sliced Swiss chard or spinach
>
> 1 cup thinly sliced red bell pepper
>
> ½ cup frozen green peas, thawed
>
> 1 cup cut fresh asparagus (1½-inch long pieces)
>
> 1½ cups cooked penne pasta

Heat the olive oil in a large, heavy saucepan over medium heat. Add the garlic and sauté 1 minute. Add the broth and thyme, and bring to a boil. Cover, reduce heat, and simmer for 10 minutes. Add the Swiss chard, bell pepper, and peas; cover and simmer 5 minutes. Add the asparagus, cover and simmer 2–4 minutes or until the asparagus is just tender.

Stir in the pasta, and cook 1 minute.

Yield: 4 servings of 2 cups each.

Nutritional Information Per Serving. Calories: 150. Energy Density: 0.4 Carbohydrate: 23 g. Fat: 3 g. Protein: 9 g. Fiber: 4 g. Sodium: 808 mg. Good Source: Folate, Vitamin C.

Asian Variation. Omit the asparagus and add 1 cup snow peas, trimmed and thinly sliced lengthwise, at the same point in the recipe. Omit pasta and add 1 cup cooked rice noodles, 1 tablespoon reduced-sodium soy sauce, and 1 teaspoon sesame oil. **Yield:** 4 servings of 2 cups each. Calories: 130.

Indian Variation. After sautéing garlic, add 2 teaspoons curry powder to the saucepan and sauté another 30 seconds, stirring constantly. Omit the pasta and add 1 cup cooked brown rice. Proceed as directed. **Yield:** 4 servings of 2 cups each. Calories: 135.

Cream of Broccoli Soup

3 cups canned low-fat or fat-free chicken broth

1½ cups fat-free evaporated milk

1 (10-ounce) package frozen chopped broccoli

1 (¾-pound) baking potato, peeled and cut into 1-inch cubes

1 cup chopped onion

½ cup sliced celery

3 cloves garlic, chopped

½ teaspoon salt

¼ teaspoon ground red pepper

Combine all the ingredients in a large, heavy saucepan, and bring to a boil over medium-high heat, stirring occasionally. Cover, reduce heat, and simmer 30 minutes, stirring occasionally.

Process the mixture, in batches, in a food processor or blender until smooth. Reheat in a saucepan. This soup can be stored in covered containers in the refrigerator for up to 3 days, or in the freezer for up to 1 month.

Yield: 7 servings of 1 cup each.

Nutritional Information Per Serving. Calories: 110. Energy Density: 0.5. Carbohydrate: 18 g. Fat: 0 g. Protein: 8 g. Fiber: 2 g. Sodium: 504 mg. Good Source: Vitamin C.

Potato Leek Soup

For a main dish, see below.

2 teaspoons canola oil

2 cups chopped leek, white and paler green parts only

½ cup chopped celery

1 bay leaf

3½ cups canned low-fat or fat-free chicken broth

2½ cups low-fat (1 percent) milk

1¾ pounds baking potatoes, peeled and cut into ¾-inch cubes

1 teaspoon paprika

½ teaspoon salt

¼ teaspoon black pepper

2 tablespoons all-purpose flour

Heat the oil in a large, heavy saucepan or Dutch oven over medium heat. Add the leek, celery, and bay leaf. Cook for 5 minutes, stirring occasionally.

Add the broth, and bring to a boil. Cover, reduce heat, and simmer for 15 minutes.

Increase the heat to medium-high, and add the milk, potatoes, paprika, salt and pepper. Bring to a boil, cover, reduce heat, and simmer for 15–20 minutes. Remove and discard the bay leaf. Drain the potato mixture, reserving the liquid and solids separately.

Place the potato mixture in the container of an electric blender, and add 1 cup of the reserved broth mixture. Add the flour to the blender, and process on low speed until smooth.

Return the mixture to the saucepan, and stir in the remaining broth. Cook over medium heat until the soup is thick and bubbly, stirring frequently.

Yield: 9 servings of 1 cup each.

Nutritional Information Per Serving. Calories: 130. Energy Density: 0.5 Carbohydrate: 24 g. Fat: 2 g. Protein: 6 g. Fiber: 2 g. Sodium: 398 mg.

Main Dish Variation. Increase the serving size to 1½ cups, and add 3 ounces (⅔ cup) diced lean ham to each serving. Cook just until hot. Calories: 311.

Vegetable Curry Soup

For main dish variations, see below.

2 teaspoons olive oil

1½ cups thinly sliced mushrooms

2 cloves garlic, minced

4 teaspoons curry powder

3½ cups canned vegetable broth

1 (14½-ounce) can Italian-style stewed tomatoes, undrained

½ cup water

2 cups diced, peeled butternut squash

1 cup thinly sliced carrot

1½ cups small cauliflowerets

1½ cups small broccoli flowerets

Heat the olive oil in a large, heavy saucepan over medium heat. Add the mushrooms and garlic, and cook for 5 minutes, stirring frequently. Add the curry powder and stir for 1 minute.

Stir in the broth, tomatoes, and water, and bring to a boil.

Add the squash and carrots, cover, and simmer for 10 minutes.

Add the cauliflowerets and broccoli flowerets; cover and simmer 10 minutes or until tender.

Yield: 5 servings of 2 cups each.

Nutritional Information Per Serving. Calories: 130. Energy Density: 0.3. Carbohydrate: 24 g. Fat: 3 g. Protein: 6 g. Fiber: 5 g. Sodium: 1,066 mg. Good Source: Fiber, Vitamin A, Vitamin C.

Main Dish Variation. For the entire recipe, add 1 pound boneless, cubed fresh sea bass, snapper, grouper, or other firm white fish during the last 5 minutes of cooking time. Serve the soup in bowls over ¾ cup cooked couscous or rice. Calories: 350.

Vegetarian Main Dish Variation. Stir 1 (19-ounce) can chickpeas (garbanzo beans) into the soup along with the cauliflower and broccoli. Serve the soup in bowls over ¾ cup cooked couscous per serving. Calories: 365.

Corn Chowder

This makes a comforting first course, or, with the addition of chicken or salmon, the centerpiece of dinner. See dinner #17 in "Menus" (p. 168), for serving suggestions.

- 3 cups canned low-fat or fat-free chicken broth
- 2¾ cups (16 ounces) lightly packed frozen hash brown potatoes, thawed
- 1 (10-ounce) package frozen whole kernel corn
- 1 cup chopped onion
- 1 cup chopped green pepper
- ½ cup finely chopped celery
- ½ teaspoon dried thyme
- 1½ cups low-fat (1 percent) milk
- 2 tablespoons all-purpose flour
- ½ teaspoons salt
- ¼ teaspoon ground red pepper

Combine the first seven ingredients in a large saucepan, and bring to a boil over medium-high heat. Cover, reduce heat, and simmer for 20 minutes.

Using a slotted spoon, transfer 2½ cups of the vegetable mixture to a food processor or blender. Process until smooth. Add the milk, flour, salt, and red pepper; process until blended. Add to the remaining vegetables in saucepan. Cook over medium heat until the soup is thick and bubbly, stirring frequently.

Serve immediately, or store in covered containers in refrigerator for up to 3 days, or in the freezer for up to 1 month.

Yield: 8 servings of 1 cup each.

Nutritional Information Per Serving. Calories: 140. Energy Density: 0.6. Carbohydrate: 27 g. Fat: 1 g. Protein: 6 g. Fiber: 3 g. Sodium: 416 mg. Good Source: Vitamin C.

Main Dish Variation. For each serving, add 3 ounces (about ⅔ cup) chopped cooked chicken breast (or white meat) or flaked canned salmon. This will increase the serving size to 2 cups. **With chicken.** Calories: 275. **With salmon.** Calories: 260.

Mushroom Barley Soup

This is a hearty first-course soup; add sirloin steak for a main dish. See dinner #15 in "Menus" (p. 168) for serving suggestions.

   3½ cups low-fat or fat-free beef broth
   1 cup water
   ½ cup pearl barley
   1 teaspoon dried thyme
   2 teaspoons olive oil
   ¾ cup finely diced carrot
   ½ cup finely diced celery
   1 (8-ounce) package presliced mushrooms
   3 medium cloves garlic, minced
   Garnish: 1 tablespoon thinly sliced green onion and
      1 tablespoon minced fresh parsley for each serving (optional)

Combine the broth, water, barley, and thyme in a large, heavy saucepan, and bring to a boil. Cover, reduce heat, and simmer 30 minutes.

   Meanwhile, heat the oil in a nonstick skillet over medium heat. Add the carrot and celery, and sauté 5 minutes. Add mushrooms and garlic, and sauté 10 minutes. Stir into the soup mixture.

   Return the soup to a boil, cover, reduce heat, and simmer 15 minutes. Remove the saucepan from the heat.

   Ladle the soup in bowls, and, if desired, sprinkle with garnish.

Yield: 4 servings of 1⅓ cups each.

Nutritional Information Per Serving. Calories: 155. Energy Density: 0.4. Carbohydrate: 26 g. Fat: 4 g. Protein: 7 g. Fiber: 5 g. Sodium: 559 mg. Good Source: Fiber, Vitamin A.

Main Dish Variation. Sauté 8 ounces of diced boneless beef sirloin in one teaspoon olive oil in the nonstick skillet over medium-high heat until the beef is browned, about 5–6 minutes, and remove the beef and juices from the saucepan. Add the beef and its juices to the beef broth, water, barley and thyme, and proceed as directed. **Yield:** 3 servings of 2⅓ cups each. Calories: 320.

Chicken, Rice, and Vegetable Soup

3½ cups canned low-fat or fat-free chicken broth

1 cup water

1 cup thinly sliced carrot

½ cup thinly sliced celery

4 cloves garlic, minced

1 teaspoon dry thyme

½ teaspoon salt

¼ teaspoon pepper

2 cups seeded and chopped plum tomatoes

1¾ cups chopped cooked white meat chicken

1 cup cooked rice

½ cup thinly sliced green onion

Combine the first eight ingredients in a large saucepan, and bring to a boil. Cover, reduce heat, and simmer 20 minutes.

Stir in the tomatoes, chicken, rice, and green onion, and simmer, covered, for 5 minutes.

Yield: 4 servings of 1¾ cups each.

Nutritional Information Per Serving. Calories: 210. Energy Density: 0.4. Carbohydrate: 22 g. Fat: 3 g. Protein: 24 g. Fiber: 3 g. Sodium: 890 mg. Good Source: Protein, Vitamin A.

Roast Turkey Soup

Fresh roasted turkey is a delicious, lean meat. This recipe yields enough for the soup, with more than enough left over for lunch the next day.

1 whole turkey breast (4–7 pounds) or 2¼ cups (12 ounces) roasted turkey breast

2 teaspoons olive oil

1 teaspoon salt

½ teaspoon pepper

4 cups canned low-fat or fat-free chicken broth

2 cups whole baby carrots

1 cup frozen pearl onions

½ cup sliced celery

1 bay leaf

10 ounces red potatoes, cut into ¾-inch cubes

1½ cups diced zucchini

Preheat the oven to 350 degrees F.

If you are roasting the turkey yourself, remove the skin and fat from the turkey breasts. Place the turkey breasts in a 13-inch x 9-inch x 2-inch baking pan. Rub each turkey breast half with 1 teaspoon olive oil, and sprinkle each with ½ teaspoon salt and ¼ teaspoon pepper.

Cover tightly with aluminum foil, and roast until the turkey releases clear juices when pricked deeply with a fork, and registers 160 degrees F. on an instant-read thermometer, about 15–20 minutes per pound. Let it cool.

Pour the chicken broth into a large, heavy saucepan or Dutch oven, add the carrots, pearl onions, celery, and bay leaf. Bring to a boil; cover, reduce heat, and simmer 15 minutes. Add the potatoes; simmer, covered, 10 minutes.

Chop enough turkey to measure 2¼ cups (12 ounces); refrigerate the rest of the turkey (use for a main dish or sandwiches). Add zucchini and chopped turkey; cover and simmer 10–15 minutes or until vegetables are tender.

Yield: 5 servings of 2 cups each.

Nutritional Information Per Serving. Calories: 205. Energy Density: 0.4. Carbohydrate: 20 g. Fat: 3 g. Protein: 25 g. Fiber: 4 g. Sodium: 575 mg. Good Source: Protein, Vitamin A, Vitamin C.

Basic Dinner Salad with Vegetables

This is a very flexible recipe. Let the freshness of the lettuces, greens, and vegetables at your market make up your mind about what goes in your salad.

> 1½ cups any combination of these salad greens: sliced romaine, torn fresh spinach, arugula, green or red leaf, mixed baby lettuces, curly endive, Boston, or Bibb.
>
> ¾ cup any combination of these vegetables: sliced onion, sliced cucumber, sliced or shredded carrot, sliced celery, sliced fennel, sliced mushrooms, broccoli flowerets, sliced cauliflowerets, cherry tomato halves or cubed tomato, sliced yellow squash or zucchini, or any vegetable from Category 1 (p. 107)

Toss the lettuces and vegetables together, and dress with 2 tablespoons Tomato Herb Vinaigrette (p. 214), Creamy Cucumber Ranch Salad Dressing (p. 212), or any low-calorie commercial salad dressing.

Yield: 1 serving.

Note: To make a salad for more people, increase the amounts of salad greens, vegetables and salad dressing according to these proportions.

Nutritional Information Per Serving. Calories: 40. Energy Density: 0.2. Carbohydrate: 7 g. Fat: 1 g. Protein: 3 g. Fiber: 3 g. Sodium: 28 mg. Good Source: Folate, Vitamin A, Vitamin C.

With Tomato Herb Dressing. Calories: 75 calories.

With Creamy Cucumber Ranch Salad Dressing. Calories: 80 calories.

Basic Dinner Salad with Fruit

Fruit is a sweet addition to a green salad.

> 1½ cups any combination of the following lettuces: sliced romaine, torn fresh spinach, arugula, green or red leaf, mixed baby lettuces, curly endive, Boston, or Bibb
>
> ¾ cup any combination of the following fruits: strawberry halves, citrus segments, pineapple cubes, apple slices, pear slices, or any fruit from Category 1 (p. 107)

Toss the lettuces and fruits together, and dress with 2 tablespoons Citrus Vinaigrette (p. 213).

Yield: 1 serving.

Note: To make a salad for more people, increase the amounts of salad greens, fruits, and salad dressing according to these proportions.

Nutritional Information Per Serving. Calories: 55. Energy Density: 0.3. Carbohydrate: 13 g. Fat: 1 g. Protein: 2 g. Fiber: 7 g. Sodium: 52 mg. Good Source: Fiber.

With Citrus Vinaigrette. Calories: 135.

Chef's Salad

4 cups lightly packed, torn fresh spinach leaves

3 cups sliced romaine lettuce leaves

1 cup alfalfa spouts

1 cup small cauliflowerets

1 cup thinly sliced red or green bell pepper

1 cup sliced fresh mushrooms

¾ cup thinly sliced carrot

2 hard-cooked eggs, chopped

4 ounces thinly sliced lean, low-salt ham, cut into thin strips

4 ounces thinly sliced part-skim mozzarella cheese, cut into thin strips

1 cup cherry tomatoes, halved

Combine the spinach, romaine, and alfalfa spouts in a large salad bowl, and toss well. Layer the cauliflowerets and the next six ingredients on top.

Add ½ cup Cucumber Ranch Salad Dressing (p. 212) or any low-calorie salad dressing, and toss well. Garnish with cherry tomatoes.

Yield: 4 servings of 1 cup each.

Note: As an alternative to ham, substitute 4 ounces roasted skinless chicken breast, cut into thin strips.

Nutritional Information Per Serving. Calories: 200. Energy Density: 0.6. Carbohydrate: 11 g. Fat: 9 g. Protein: 19 g. Fiber: 6 g. Sodium: 628 mg. Good Source: Protein, Fiber, Folate, Vitamin C.

With Cucumber Ranch Dressing. Calories: 240.

Crunchy and Creamy Potato Salad

¼ cup fat-free sour cream

¼ cup low-fat or fat-free buttermilk

¼ cup reduced-fat mayonnaise

1½ tablespoons reduced-calorie ranch-style salad dressing mix

1½ pounds medium-size red potatoes (about 5)

3 tablespoons tarragon vinegar

¼ teaspoon salt

1 medium cucumber

1 cup cherry tomatoes, quartered

½ cup diced celery

½ cup diced red or green bell pepper

⅓ cup mixed minced fresh herbs: parsley, chives, dill or basil

Combine the first four ingredients in a small bowl, and mix well. Cover and refrigerate.

In a large saucepan, place the potatoes, cover them with water, and bring to a boil. Reduce heat, and simmer, partially covered, for 20–25 minutes or until tender.

Drain in a colander, and let cool slightly. Cut the potatoes into ¼-inch-thick slices, and toss with vinegar and salt in a large bowl. Let cool completely, tossing occasionally.

Cut the cucumber in half lengthwise and slice it thin. Add the cucumber, tomatoes, celery, bell pepper, and herbs to potatoes. Toss gently with the dressing. Cover and refrigerate at least 1 hour.

Yield: 8 servings of ¾ cup each.

Note: You can store this covered in the refrigerator for up to 3 days.

Nutritional Information Per Serving. Calories: 105. Energy Density: 0.7. Carbohydrate: 20 g. Fat: 2 g. Protein: 2 g. Fiber: 2 g. Sodium: 217 mg.

Moroccan Garden Couscous

This couscous salad is made more *Volumetric* with a generous selection of vegetables.

1 tablespoon olive oil

1 cup chopped onion

2 large cloves garlic, minced

½ teaspoon ground ginger

½ teaspoon ground cumin

½ teaspoon ground turmeric

2½ cups canned vegetable broth

½ teaspoon salt

1 cup baby carrots, cut in half, lengthwise

1½ cups (6 ounces) fresh green beans, trimmed and cut in half

1¼ cups red or green bell peppers, sliced into 1½-inch pieces

1½ cups sliced zucchini

1 cup couscous, uncooked

½ cup seeded and diced plum tomato

¼ cup minced cilantro

Heat the olive oil in a large heavy skillet over medium heat. Add the onion and garlic, and sauté until tender, about 5 minutes. Stir in the ginger, cumin, and turmeric, and sauté 1 minute.

Pour in the broth, add the salt, and bring to a boil. Add the carrots, beans, and pepper; cover, reduce heat, and simmer 5 minutes. Add the zucchini, and simmer, covered, 5 minutes.

Uncover, increase the heat to medium-high heat. When the mixture boils, stir in the couscous. Cover, remove the skillet from the heat, and let it stand for 5 minutes.

Stir in the tomato and cilantro, fluffing with a fork.

Yield: 4 servings of 1½ cups each.

Nutritional Information Per Serving. Calories: 290. Energy Density: 0.7. Carbohydrate: 53 g. Fat: 5 g. Protein: 10 g. Fiber: 7 g. Sodium: 960 mg. Good Source: Fiber, Vitamin C.

Waldorf Salad

½ cup water

¼ cup fresh lemon juice, divided

2 firm, ripe pears or apples

1 Granny Smith or Red Delicious apple

3 ribs celery, split lengthwise and cut into ½-inch pieces (½ cup)

1 cup seedless red or green grapes, halved

2 tablespoons finely minced walnuts, toasted

⅔ cup low-fat or fat-free vanilla-flavored yogurt

2 tablespoons low-fat mayonnaise

2 teaspoons sugar

Combine the water with 2 tablespoons of the lemon juice in a medium bowl. Working with one piece of fruit at a time, core and dice pears and apple, and toss with the water mixture. Refrigerate for 10 minutes.

Drain the fruit well, place it in a large bowl, add the celery, grapes, and walnuts, and toss gently.

Combine the yogurt, mayonnaise, the remaining 2 tablespoons of lemon juice and the sugar, and pour over the fruit mixture. Toss. Cover and chill at least 1 hour before serving.

Yield: 4 servings of 1 cup each.

Note: You can keep this, covered, in the refrigerator up to 24 hours.

Nutritional Information Per Serving. Calories: 170. Energy Density: 0.7 Carbohydrate: 35 g. Fat: 3 g. Protein: 3 g. Fiber: 4 g. Sodium: 119 mg.

Fruit Salad

2 cups seedless grape halves, halved

2 cups fresh strawberry halves

2 cups sliced fresh or frozen, thawed peaches

2 cups cantaloupe cubes or melon balls

½ cup vanilla-flavored low-fat or fat-free yogurt

3 tablespoons frozen orange juice concentrate, thawed

1 tablespoon sugar

¼ teaspoon ground cinnamon, optional

Combine the fruit in a bowl or a food storage container; refrigerate. This will keep up to 24 hours.

In a small bowl, mix the yogurt, orange juice concentrate, sugar, and, if desired, cinnamon. This, too, can be made in advance and refrigerated for up to 24 hours.

For each serving, toss 1 cup of the fruit mixture with 1½ tablespoons of the yogurt mixture.

Yield: 8 servings of 1 heaping cup each.

Nutritional Information Per Serving. Calories: 110. Energy Density: 0.5. Carbohydrate: 26 g. Fat: 1 g. Protein: 2 g. Fiber: 3 g. Sodium: 16 mg. Good Source: Vitamin C.

Fruit Salad Mold

Fruit in aspic was once the height of culinary fashion. It's a tradition worth revisiting. Serve this as a refreshing side dish with dinner, as a snack, or as dessert.

2 (0.3-ounce) packages sugar-free strawberry-flavored gelatin
2 cups boiling water
1½ cups cold water
1 (15½-ounce) can pineapple tidbits in unsweetened juice, undrained
1 (11-ounce) can mandarin oranges, drained
1½ cups seedless green grape halves
½ cup finely diced celery

In a large bowl, dissolve the gelatin in the boiling water. Stir in the cold water, pineapple tidbits with their juice, mandarin oranges, grapes, and celery. Pour into a 2-quart mold or bowl coated with cooking spray.

Cover and refrigerate, stirring after about 30 minutes, or when it becomes the consistency of unbeaten egg whites. Refrigerate for 4 hours, or until chilled and set.

Yield: 10 servings of ¾ cup each.

Nutritional Information Per Serving. Calories: 55. Energy Density: 0.3. Carbohydrate: 13 g. Fat: 0 g. Protein: 1 g. Fiber: 1 g. Sodium: 53 mg.

Caesar Salad Dressing

2 cloves garlic, halved

⅓ cup reduced-calorie mayonnaise

¼ cup fat-free sour cream

¼ cup low-fat or fat-free buttermilk

3 tablespoons Parmesan cheese

3 tablespoons red wine vinegar

1½ tablespoons Dijon mustard

2 teaspoons Worcestershire sauce

¾ teaspoon Cajun seasoning

Process all the ingredients in a blender until smooth.

Store in a covered container in the refrigerator at least 1 hour before serving, and up to 1 week.

Yield: 1 cup (16 tablespoons).

Nutritional Information Per Tablespoon. Calories: 25. Energy Density: 1.4. Carbohydrate: 2 g. Fat: 2 g. Protein: 1 g. Fiber: 0 g. Sodium: 70 mg.

Creamy Cucumber Ranch Salad Dressing

¾ cup low-fat or fat-free buttermilk

½ cup reduced-calorie mayonnaise

1 tablespoon extra virgin olive oil

3 tablespoons minced green onion

3 tablespoons minced cilantro or fresh dill
  (or 1 teaspoon dried dill)

1 tablespoon lemon juice

½ teaspoon salt

¼ teaspoon ground red pepper

½ small cucumber, peeled and finely chopped

Combine all the ingredients in a bowl, and stir well. Pour into a covered jar.

Refrigerate at least 1 hour, and up to 4 days.

Yield: 1¾ cups (28 tablespoons).

Nutritional Information Per Tablespoon. Calories: 20. Energy Density: 1.2. Carbohydrate: 1 g. Fat: 2 g. Protein: 0 g. Fiber: 0g. Sodium: 79 mg.

Citrus Vinaigrette

¼ cup orange juice

2 tablespoons sherry vinegar

2 tablespoons extra virgin olive oil

1 tablespoon water

1 tablespoon honey

¼ teaspoon salt

¼ teaspoon pepper

Combine all the ingredients in a jar, cover tightly, and shake to blend.

Use immediately, or refrigerate up to 5 days.

Yield: ½ cup plus 2 tablespoons (10 tablespoons)

Nutritional Information Per Tablespoon. Calories: 40. Energy Density: 2.5. Carbohydrate: 4 g. Fat: 3 g. Protein: 0 g. Fiber: 0 g. Sodium: 47 mg.

Tomato Herb Vinaigrette

1½ cups peeled and finely chopped firm, ripe tomatoes

¼ cup minced green onion or chives

2 tablespoons minced fresh basil, dill, or tarragon (or 1 teaspoon dried herbs)

1 large clove garlic, finely minced

½ teaspoon sugar

½ teaspoon salt

¼ teaspoon freshly ground pepper

¼ cup balsamic vinegar

2 tablespoons extra virgin olive oil

1 tablespoon Dijon mustard

Combine the tomatoes, green onion, basil, garlic, sugar, salt, and pepper in a medium bowl, and stir well. Cover and let stand at room temperature 1 hour.

Add the vinegar, olive oil, and mustard, and stir well. Pour into a covered container. Refrigerate at least 1 hour and up to 5 days.

Yield: 1½ cups (24 tablespoons)

Nutritional Information Per Tablespoon. Calories: 20. Energy Density: 1.0. Carbohydrate: 2 g. Fat: 1 g. Protein: 0 g. Fiber: 0 g. Sodium: 52 mg.

Steak and Vegetable Kabobs

1 pound lean boneless beef sirloin, cut 1 inch thick, trimmed of fat

⅓ cup reduced-sodium soy sauce

¼ cup rice wine, sake, or rice wine vinegar

2 cloves garlic, minced

2 teaspoons sugar

2 teaspoons sesame oil

8 ounces medium to large mushrooms (about 12), stems removed

1 large red or yellow bell pepper, cut into 16 equal pieces

1 large zucchini, cut in 1-inch slices

Cut the beef into cubes and place into a medium bowl.

Pour the soy sauce, wine, garlic, sugar, and sesame oil into the container of a blender and process until blended. Pour the marinade over the beef, tossing to coat. Cover and refrigerate 1 hour, stirring occasionally.

If using wooden skewers, soak these in water 1 hour. Prepare a charcoal fire or preheat the gas grill.

Drain the meat, reserving the marinade in a small saucepan. Boil the marinade for 2 minutes; reserve for basting.

On the skewers, alternate pieces of meat, mushrooms, peppers, and zucchini. Grill kebabs about 3–4 inches from hot coals for 4–5 minutes on each side, basting occasionally with the reserved marinade.

Yield: 4 servings.

Nutritional Information Per Serving. Calories: 300. Energy Density: 1.5.
Carbohydrate: 12 g. Fat: 16 g. Protein: 27 g. Fiber: 2 g. Sodium: 725.
Good Source: Protein, Fiber, Vitamin A, Vitamin C, Iron.

Beef Stroganoff

1 (¾-pound) beef flank steak, trimmed

3 tablespoons all-purpose flour, divided

1 tablespoon mild paprika

¼ teaspoon salt

¼ teaspoon freshly ground pepper

1 tablespoon olive oil

2 cloves garlic, minced

1½ cups thinly sliced onion (about 1 large), separated into rings

1½ cups thin green pepper strips, cut 1½–2 inches long

1 (8-ounce) package presliced mushrooms

1 cup canned low-fat or fat-free beef broth

½ cup fat-free sour cream

2 cups cooked egg noodles, cooked without salt or fat

Cut the steak diagonally across the grain into thin slices.

Combine 2 tablespoons flour with the paprika, salt, and pepper in a shallow bowl; add steak and toss to coat.

Heat the olive oil in a large nonstick skillet over medium-high heat. Add the steak; cook until slices are browned on both sides, about 5 minutes. Add the garlic, onion, and green pepper; cook 2 minutes, stirring frequently. Add the mushrooms and cook uncovered for 2 minutes. Stir in the broth; bring to a boil. Cover, reduce heat to medium-low, and simmer 10 minutes.

Meanwhile, in a small bowl or cup, stir together the sour cream and the remaining 1 tablespoon flour until smooth. Stir into simmering mixture; cook, stirring constantly, 2 minutes or until thickened.

Yield: 4 servings of 1 cup each, over ½ cup noodles each.

Nutritional Information Per Serving. Calories: 395. Energy Density: 1.6. Carbohydrate: 42 g. Fat: 13 g. Protein: 29 g. Fiber: 4 g. Sodium: 383 mg. Good Source: Protein, Iron.

Great American *Volumetric* Burger

If you like a plump, juicy hamburger, this one's for you. Each sandwich weighs in at more than a half-pound, yet has only about 400 calories. See next page for a Mexican Chili Burger variation. (For a Vegetarian Burger, see p. 232.)

⅓ cup uncooked bulgur

½ cup boiling water

2 teaspoons olive oil

1 cup minced red onion

½ teaspoon sugar

1 teaspoon balsamic vinegar

¾ pound very lean ground beef or turkey

1 large clove garlic, crushed

¾ cup finely grated carrot, lightly packed

2 teaspoons Worcestershire sauce

½ teaspoon salt

½ teaspoon freshly ground pepper

4 (1½-ounce) hamburger buns

4 large leaves Boston or Bibb lettuce

4 red onion slices

4 (⅓-ounce) slices large tomato

½ cup boiling water

Optional condiments per serving: 1 tablespoon commercial fat-free blue cheese or ranch salad dressing; 1 tablespoon fat-free mayonnaise dressing; 2 teaspoons mustard; 2 teaspoons ketchup; 3 dill pickle slices; 2 pitted ripe olives, sliced.

Stir together the bulgur and ½ cup boiling water in a small bowl; let stand 30 minutes or until water is absorbed and bulgur is tender.

Meanwhile, in a nonstick skillet, heat the olive oil over medium heat. Add the onion and sugar; sauté until the onion is lightly browned, about 10 minutes. Stir in the vinegar; sauté about 20 seconds, stirring until vinegar evaporates. Remove the skillet from the heat.

In a small bowl, mix the plumped bulgur, onion mixture, beef, carrot, garlic, Worcestershire sauce, salt, and pepper.

Shape into four ¾-inch-thick patties.

Grill or broil the burger patties on a rack sprayed with vegetable cooking spray until browned and cooked, about 5 minutes per side. Arrange lettuce, tomato, and onion slices on bottom halves of buns, add the burger, add desired condiment, and serve immediately.

Yield: 4 servings.

Nutritional Information Per Serving. Calories: 400. Energy Density: 1.7. Carbohydrate: 39 g. Fat: 17 g. Protein: 22 g. Fiber: 5 g. Sodium: 652 mg. Good Source: Protein, Iron, Vitamin B–12.

Note: The fat-free blue cheese or ranch dressing adds 25 calories per serving; the ketchup, mustard, pickles, and olives each add 10 calories.

Mexican Chili Burger Variation. Omit the onion mixture. Combine the plumped bulgur mixture with the water, beef, garlic, carrot, Worcestershire sauce, salt, and pepper as directed above; add 1 cup very finely chopped plum tomato, ¼ cup minced cilantro, 1 teaspoon chili powder, and 1 teaspoon hot sauce. Form patties and cook as directed above. Arrange lettuce, tomato, and onion slices on the buns; spoon 1 tablespoon salsa and reduced-fat sour cream on each burger. Calories: 370.

Chili Ranchero

"Wet" dishes, like chili, are naturally low in energy density. We use cocoa powder for a richer taste. For a vegetarian version, see below.

½ pound very lean ground beef

2 cups chopped onion

1½ cups chopped green pepper

2 large cloves garlic, minced

2 tablespoons chili powder

2 teaspoons unsweetened cocoa powder

1 teaspoon ground cumin

½ teaspoon salt

1 (14½-ounce) can beef broth, undiluted

1 (14½-ounce) can chili-flavored chunky tomatoes, undrained

1 cup water

1 (15-ounce) can pinto beans, rinsed and drained

1 cup frozen whole kernel corn, thawed

¼ cup minced cilantro

Hot sauce to taste

Coat a large, heavy saucepan with vegetable cooking spray; place over medium-high heat until hot. Crumble beef into the saucepan, and cook until the meat loses its pink color. Stir to break up the meat. Drain in a colander.

Wipe the saucepan with paper towels, coat with cooking spray again, and place over medium-high heat until hot. Add the onion, green pepper, and garlic; sauté until tender, about 10 minutes.

Add the chili powder, cocoa powder, cumin, and salt; cook, stirring constantly, 1 minute.

Add the beef, broth, tomatoes, and water; bring to a boil.

Cover, reduce heat, and simmer 15 minutes.

Uncover and stir in beans and corn; simmer 5 additional minutes. Stir in the cilantro and hot sauce to taste.

Yield: 4 servings of 2 cups each.

Nutritional Information Per Serving. Calories: 330. Energy Density: 0.7. Carbohydrate: 40 g. Fat: 11 g. Protein: 21 g. Fiber: 10 g. Sodium: 1,130 mg. Good Source: Fiber, Vitamin C.

Vegetarian Variation. Omit the ground beef; reduce the amount of pinto beans to 1 cup. Add 1 cup canned black beans and 1 cup canned garbanzo beans; stir these into the chili at the same time that the pinto beans and corn are added. **Yield:** 4 servings of 2 cups each. Calories: 290.

Pork with Sweet Potatoes and Apples

Sweet potatoes and apples are classic partners to pork, and they boost the volume of each serving with few calories.

3 tablespoons all-purpose flour, divided

½ teaspoon salt

¼ teaspoon pepper

¾ pound pork tenderloin, cut into ¼-inch-thick slices

1 tablespoon olive oil

1 cup chopped onion

¾ cup apple cider

¾ cup canned low-fat or fat-free chicken broth

4 clove garlic, minced

1 large or 2 small sweet potatoes (a little over ½ pound), peeled and cut into ½-inch-thick slices

2 Granny Smith or small Red Delicious apples, cored and cut into ½-inch wedges

Combine 2 tablespoons of the flour with the salt and pepper in a shallow dish; dredge the pork in flour mixture.

Heat the olive oil in a large Dutch oven or deep skillet over medium-high heat. Add the pork and onion, and sauté until the pork is browned on both sides, about 2 minutes on each side. Remove from heat, and set aside.

Combine the cider with the remaining 1 tablespoon flour and stir until smooth.

Add the cider mixture, broth, garlic, sweet potato slices, and apple slices to the skillet with the pork; return to medium-high heat and bring to a boil. Cover, reduce heat, and simmer 20 minutes.

Yield: 4 servings of 1 cup each.

Nutritional Information Per Serving. Calories: 320. Energy Density: 1.3. Carbohydrate: 39 g. Fat: 6 g. Protein: 23 g. Fiber: 6 g. Sodium: 464 mg. Good Source: Protein, Iron, Fiber.

Stir-fry

A stir-fry is a quick way to create a dish that combines plenty of vegetables with lean sources of protein. The vegetables release water as they come into contact with high heat, so you don't need to add much oil to keep them from sticking, and in the later part of cooking you're actually steaming the food. You can make this dish with pork tenderloin, lean flank steak, chicken breasts, or tofu.

- ¾ pound pork tenderloin, ¾ pound lean flank steak, ¾ pound skinned and boned chicken breast halves, or 8 ounces firm tofu
- 1 tablespoon dark sesame oil, divided
- 1½ tablespoons minced peeled fresh ginger
- 3 cloves garlic, chopped
- ½ cup beef broth
- 3 tablespoons low-sodium soy sauce
- 1 tablespoon cornstarch
- 1 cup bell pepper strips, green, red, or yellow
- 1 cup small broccoli florets
- 1 cup diagonally sliced carrot
- ½ cup drained, canned water chestnuts
- ½ cup drained, canned bamboo shoots
- 1 cup fresh bean sprouts
- 3 cups cooked rice (optional)

Cut the pork, beef, chicken into 2-inch x 1¼-inch strips; if using tofu, cut into ¾-inch cubes. Toss with 2 teaspoons sesame oil, ginger, and garlic in a medium bowl. Cover and let stand 10 minutes.

Combine the beef broth, soy sauce, and cornstarch in a small bowl, and stir until smooth and set aside.

Heat a large, nonstick skillet over medium-high heat; add the pork (or beef, chicken, or tofu) mixture, and sauté until browned, about 5 minutes. Remove from the skillet, and transfer to a plate.

Add the remaining 1 teaspoon sesame oil to skillet, and toss in pepper strips, broccoli, carrot, water chestnuts, and bamboo shoots. Stir-fry 3–4 minutes or until the vegetables are crisp-tender. Stir the broth mixture and pour into the skillet; stir well. Add the cooked pork (or beef, chicken or tofu); stir in bean sprouts.

Cook, stirring constantly, 1–2 minutes or until mixture is hot and thickened. Serve over rice, if desired.

Yield: 4 servings of 1¼ cups each.

Nutritional Information Per Serving (with Pork). Calories: 215. Energy Density: 1.0. Carbohydrate: 17 g. Fat: 6 g. Protein: 24 g. Fiber: 4 g. Sodium: 601 mg. Good Source: Vitamin A, Vitamin C.

With rice. 365 calories.

With flank steak. Calories: 250. Calories with rice: 400.

With chicken breast. Calories: 203. Calories with rice: 355.

With tofu. Calories: 155. Calories with rice: 300. (Note: Tofu is so low in energy density that you can increase the serving size of this version to 2 cups for 250 calories; with rice it's 400 calories.)

Calypso Chicken Packages

Baking chicken breast with black beans, corn, and pineapple fills your plate with a succulent, spicy main dish.

12 ounces skinned and boned chicken breast halves

1 (15-ounce) can pineapple chunks in unsweetened juice, undrained

¾ cup rinsed and drained canned black beans

¾ cup frozen whole kernel corn

¼ cup chopped cilantro

2 teaspoons chili powder

½ teaspoon salt

¼ teaspoon ground red pepper

3 cups hot, cooked rice (optional)

Preheat the oven to 350 degrees F.

Cut the chicken into 1-inch strips; place in a large bowl.

Drain the pineapple, reserving 3 tablespoons juice.

In a large bowl, combine the drained pineapple and reserved pineapple juice with the black beans, corn, cilantro, chili powder, salt, red pepper, and chicken. Toss well.

Tear off four 10-inch pieces of heavy-duty aluminum foil, and mound the chicken mixture into the center of each foil piece; fold the foil over mixture and seal well. (You can use foil baking bags as an alternative.)

Place on a baking sheet. Bake 35–40 minutes or until chicken is cooked (no pink inside; juices run clear). Unwrap and serve.

Yield: 4 servings.

Note: To serve over rice, cook 3 cups; that allows ¾ cup per person.

Nutritional Information Per Serving. Calories: 250. Energy Density: 0.8. Carbohydrate: 23 g. Fat: 4 g. Protein: 31 g. Fiber: 5 g. Sodium: 358 mg. Good Source: Protein, Iron.

With ¾ cup rice. Calories: 400.

Chicken Pot Pie

A conventional pot pie, with crust on the outside and cream inside, is one comfort food that can widen waists. This one is lighter, without a crust, but topped with fresh, warm biscuits.

2 teaspoons olive oil

2 cups sliced mushrooms

1½ cups chopped leek

3 cloves garlic, minced

4¾ cups canned low-fat or fat-free chicken broth, divided

1½ cups thinly sliced carrot

1 cup chopped green pepper

¾ cup diced celery

¼ cup all-purpose flour

2⅓ cups chopped cooked white meat chicken (1 pound)

½ teaspoon freshly ground pepper

1 cup reduced-fat biscuit baking mix

¼ cup plus 3 tablespoons low-fat (1 percent) milk

Preheat the oven to 400 degrees F.

Heat the olive oil in a large heavy saucepan over medium heat. Add the mushrooms, leek, and garlic; sauté 5 minutes. Add 4¼ cups chicken broth, carrot, green pepper, and celery; bring to a boil. Cover, reduce heat, and simmer 5 minutes or until vegetables are just tender.

In a cup, stir together the flour and remaining ½ cup chicken broth until smooth; stir into broth mixture. Add the chicken and pepper; bring to a boil, stirring constantly. Pour into a shallow 1½- or 2-quart baking dish coated with vegetable cooking spray.

Stir together the baking mix and milk to make a soft dough. Drop the biscuit topping by heaping tablespoonfuls onto the chicken mixture to form 10 biscuits.

Bake 20–25 minutes or until the biscuits are golden.

Yield: 5 servings of 1⅓ cups each.

Nutritional Information Per Serving. Calories: 305. Energy Density: 0.9. Carbohydrate: 34 g. Fat: 7 g. Protein: 28 g. Fiber: 3 g. Sodium: 988 mg. Good Source: Protein, Iron.

Peanut Chicken Stew

1 teaspoon canola oil

1 cup chopped onion

2 cloves garlic, minced

¾ pound skinned and boned chicken breast halves, cut into 1-inch
cubes

3½ cups canned low-fat or fat-free chicken broth

¾ pound sweet potatoes, peeled and cut into ½-inch cubes

1½ cups cut fresh green beans

2 cups sliced fresh spinach

¾ cup diced red bell pepper

3 tablespoons reduced-fat smooth peanut butter

2 tablespoons lemon juice

Hot sauce to taste

Garnishes: 1 tablespoon each sliced green onion, minced cilantro,
finely chopped unsalted dry roasted peanuts per serving
(optional)

Heat oil in a large saucepan over medium-high heat. Add onion and
garlic; sauté 4 minutes or until tender. Add chicken; cook until chicken
loses its pink color, stirring frequently. Add broth, sweet potatoes, and
beans to saucepan; bring to a boil. Cover, reduce heat, and simmer
10–15 minutes or until vegetables are tender. Stir in spinach and red
bell pepper; cover and simmer 5 minutes. Stir in peanut butter, lemon
juice, and hot sauce until blended; simmer 1 minute. Remove from
heat, and ladle into bowls. Sprinkle with toppings, if desired.

Yield: 4 servings of 1¾ cups each.

Nutritional Information Per Serving. Calories: 330. Energy Density: 0.8.
Carbohydrate: 39 g. Fat: 7 g. Protein: 29 g. Fiber: 7g. Sodium: 708 mg.
Good Source: Protein, Fiber, Vitamin C.

Main Dish Variation. Ladle each serving over ½ cup cooked rice.
Calories: 435.

Chicken and Fruit Salad

½ cup fat-free plain yogurt

½ cup fat-free mayonnaise or salad dressing

1 tablespoon frozen orange juice concentrate, thawed

¼ teaspoon ground ginger

⅛ teaspoon ground red pepper

⅓ cup thinly sliced green onion

1½ cups seedless red or green grapes, halved

1½ cups thinly sliced celery

1½ cups chopped cooked chicken (½ pound)

½ cup chopped water chestnuts

4 large leaf lettuce leaves

2 plum tomatoes, thinly sliced

1 cucumber, thinly sliced

Combine the first five ingredients in a medium bowl; stir in the green onion.

Combine the grapes, celery, chicken, and water chestnuts in a large bowl. Toss well with the dressing. Cover and refrigerate 2–4 hours.

To serve, line each salad plate with a lettuce leaf, and arrange one-fourth of the tomatoes and cucumber slices on top of lettuce. Spoon one-fourth of the chicken mixture on top.

Yield: 4 servings of 1¼ cups each, plus the lettuce, tomato, and cucumber slices.

Nutritional Information Per Serving. Calories: 200. Energy Density: 0.5. Carbohydrate: 24 g. Fat: 2 g. Protein: 19 g. Fiber: 3 g. Sodium: 351 mg. Good Source: Protein, Vitamin C.

Baked Red Snapper Provençale

Red snapper baked in broth or wine, with tomatoes and zucchini, yields a dish that is aromatic, moist, delicious, and very low in calories. Or substitute any lean, white fish fillets.

    1 tablespoon olive oil
    1½ cups chopped onion
    2 cups chopped seeded plum tomato
    2 cloves garlic, minced
    1 bay leaf
    ¼ cup canned low-fat or fat-free chicken broth, or dry white wine
    ¼ cup minced fresh basil or 1 teaspoon dried basil
    ¼ teaspoon salt
    ¼ teaspoon pepper
    4 (4-ounce) snapper or grouper fillets
    2 cups thinly sliced zucchini (about 2 medium)
    1 bell pepper, thinly sliced

Preheat the oven to 350 degrees F.

Heat the olive oil in a 2-quart saucepan over medium heat. Add the chopped onion; sauté until tender. Add the chopped tomato, garlic, bay leaf, wine, basil, salt, and pepper. Cover, reduce heat to medium-low, and simmer 10 minutes, stirring occasionally.

Arrange the fish fillets in a single layer in a 11-inch x 7-inch or shallow 2-quart baking dish coated with vegetable cooking spray. Sprinkle fillets evenly with ¼ teaspoon salt. Arrange the zucchini and pepper slices on and around fish. Spoon the tomato sauce evenly over the fish and vegetables.

Cover and bake 30–40 minutes or until the fish flakes with a fork.

Yield: 4 servings.

Nutritional Information Per Serving. Calories: 240. Energy Density: 0.8. Carbohydrate: 17 g. Fat: 6 g. Protein: 32 g. Fiber: 4 g. Sodium: 398 mg. Good Source: Protein, Vitamin C.

Shrimp and Vegetable Risotto

This is a rich, comforting dish.

4 teaspoons olive oil, divided

1½ cups cut fresh green beans (½-inch pieces)

1½ cups finely diced carrot

¾ cup finely chopped onion

3 cups lightly packed chopped fresh spinach

1 cup sugar snap peas or snow peas, trimmed and sliced crosswise
   into ½-inch pieces

16 medium shrimp, peeled, deveined, and halved lengthwise

¼ teaspoon salt

1 (14½-ounce) can low-fat or fat-free chicken broth

1½ cups water

1 cup Arborio rice, uncooked

½ teaspoon salt

¼ teaspoon freshly ground pepper

⅓ cup freshly grated Romano cheese

Heat 2 teaspoons olive oil in a large, heavy saucepan over medium-
high heat. Add the green beans, carrot, and onion, and sauté 10 minutes or until just tender.

Add the spinach and sugar snap peas, cover, and cook 3 minutes.

Stir in the shrimp and ¼ teaspoon salt; cover and cook 1 minute.
Transfer mixture to a bowl, and set aside.

In a small saucepan, simmer the broth and water, but do not boil.
Keep warm over low heat.

In a large, clean saucepan, heat the remaining 2 teaspoons olive oil
over medium-high heat, and add the rice. Cook 2 minutes, stirring constantly. Pour in 1½ cups hot broth mixture; reduce heat to medium,
and cook until liquid is nearly absorbed, stirring occasionally (about
8–10 minutes).

Add the remaining broth mixture in three batches, stirring constantly until each portion of broth is absorbed before adding the next
(about 20 minutes total cooking time).

Stir in the vegetable and shrimp mixture, ¼ teaspoon salt and pepper; cook 3 minutes or until hot. Stir in cheese. Serve immediately.

Yield: 4 servings of 1¼ cups each.

Nutritional Information Per Serving. Calories: 360. Energy Density: 1.1.
Carbohydrate: 55 g. Fat: 7 g. Protein: 16 g. Fiber: 5 g. Sodium: 582 mg.
Good Source: Protein, Vitamin A.

Tuna Ranch Salad

⅓ cup Creamy Cucumber Ranch Salad Dressing (page 212)
2 tablespoons minced fresh basil or tarragon (optional)
1 garlic clove, minced
1 (9-ounce) can chunk water-packed white tuna, drained and flaked
½ cup finely diced celery
½ cup grated carrot
⅓ cup thinly sliced green onion
¼ cup finely chopped pitted ripe olives (optional)
2 large tomatoes (about 1 pound)
4 leaf lettuce leaves
Freshly ground pepper

Combine the salad dressing, basil, and garlic and mix well.

Combine the tuna, celery, carrot, green onion, and olives, and toss with the salad dressing. Cover and refrigerate 1 hour or until serving time. (Can be stored, covered, up to 3 days at this stage.)

Just before serving, cut each tomato into 6 wedges, beginning at the stem end and cutting to within ½ inch from the opposite end. Open each tomato gently, and place it on a lettuce-lined serving plate. Spoon the tuna mixture evenly into the tomatoes, and sprinkle with pepper.

Yield: 2 servings of 1¼ cups each.

Nutritional Information Per Serving. Calories: 300. Energy Density: 0.6.
Carbohydrate: 21 g. Fat: 10 g. Protein: 34 g. Fiber: 5 g. Sodium: 741 mg.
Good Source: Protein, Fiber, Vitamin C.

With olives: 319 calories.

Volumetric Pizza

This pizza is such a good illustration of methods to lower energy density that we've illustrated it in "Modifying Favorite Recipes" (p. 255).

   2 tablespoons cornmeal
   1 (10-ounce) can refrigerated pizza dough
   1½ cups small broccoli florets
   1 cup sliced cauliflowerets
   1 (14½-ounce) can diced tomatoes with garlic and basil, drained
   1 cup thin, 2-inch-long strips red or green bell pepper
   ½ cup thinly sliced mushrooms
   ½ cup diced yellow squash or zucchini
   ½ small onion, vertically sliced into thin slices (about ½ cup)
   1½ cups (6 ounces) shredded part-skim mozzarella cheese
   4½ ounces Canadian bacon (optional)
   ¼ cup grated Parmesan cheese

Preheat the oven to 425 degrees F.

Coat a 12-inch pizza pan or 12-inch x 8-inch baking pan with vegetable cooking spray; sprinkle with cornmeal. Unroll the pizza dough and place it in the pan. Starting at center, press out dough to edges of pan using your hands. Bake 5 minutes or until crust just begins to brown.

Meanwhile, microwave the broccoli and cauliflower in a large glass bowl with 3 tablespoons water, covered, at high power for 2–3 minutes or until crisp-tender, stirring once. Drain well.

Pulse the tomatoes in a food processor just until crushed. Take the pizza crust out of the oven, and spoon the tomato mixture evenly on it. Top with cooked broccoli and cauliflower; sprinkle with bell pepper, mushrooms, squash, and onion. If desired, top with Canadian bacon. Combine mozzarella and Parmesan cheese; sprinkle over the pizza.

Bake 11–15 minutes or until crust is golden brown and vegetables are hot. With a serrated knife or pizza cutter, cut into 6 slices.

Yield: 6 servings.

Nutritional Information Per Serving. Calories: 270. Energy Density: 2.4. Carbohydrate: 37 g. Fat: 8 g. Protein: 15 g. Fiber: 5 g. Sodium: 771 mg. Good Source: Fiber, Vitamin A, Folate.

With Canadian bacon. Calories: 290.

Four-Cheese Vegetable Lasagna

Lasagna can be a heavy, caloric dish. This one is both flavorful and lighter. With plenty of vegetables, the energy density plummets, which allows this tasty version to be made with real Parmesan cheese and lower-fat cheeses, rather than fat-free cheeses, and still provide nearly ½ pound per serving for under 250 calories.

12 uncooked lasagna noodles, cooked and drained

2 teaspoons olive oil

2 cups chopped broccoli

2 cups sliced mushrooms

1½ cups thinly sliced carrot

½ cup chopped red or green bell pepper

3 cloves garlic, minced

1 cup sliced green onion

½ teaspoon salt

½ teaspoon freshly ground pepper

2 cups low-fat (1 percent) cottage cheese

1 cup (4 ounces) shredded part-skim mozzarella cheese

¾ cup (3 ounces) shredded reduced-fat Jarlsberg cheese or part-skim Swiss cheese

1 (10-ounce) package frozen chopped spinach, thawed and squeezed dry

2 cups commercial fat-free spaghetti sauce

¼ cup grated Parmesan cheese

Cook the lasagna noodles according to the package directions, omitting salt and fat. Drain and set aside. (If you are using "no-cook" noodles, omit this step.)

Preheat the oven to 375 degrees F.

Heat the olive oil in a large, deep skillet or Dutch oven over medium-high heat until hot. Add the broccoli and the next five ingredients; sauté about 5 minutes. Stir in ¼ teaspoon salt and ¼ teaspoon pepper. Set aside.

Combine the cottage cheese, mozzarella cheese, Jarlsberg cheese, and spinach in a large bowl; add ¼ teaspoon salt and ¼ teaspoon pepper. Mix thoroughly.

Spread ½ cup tomato sauce on bottom of a 13-inch x 9-inch x 2-inch baking dish coated with vegetable cooking spray. Arrange 4 lasagna noodles over the sauce. Top with half the cottage cheese mixture, half the broccoli mixture, and half the remaining spaghetti sauce. Repeat layers, and end with a layer of noodles. Spoon the remaining ½ cup spaghetti sauce on the noodles; sprinkle evenly with Parmesan cheese.

Cover with aluminum foil and bake 45 minutes. Let stand 10 minutes before serving. Slice in half lengthwise, then in five equal widths.

Yield: 10 servings.

Nutritional Information Per Serving. Calories: 245. Energy Density: 1.1. Carbohydrate: 30 g. Fat: 6 g. Protein: 18 g. Fiber: 3 g. Sodium: 562 mg. Good Source: Protein, Calcium, Vitamin A, Vitamin C.

Vegetarian Burger

Frozen veggie burgers are okay, but once you've tasted this fresh version, you'll be hooked.

½ cup bulgur, uncooked

⅔ cup boiling water

2 teaspoons olive oil

2 tablespoons minced walnuts

2 teaspoons ground cumin

1 (15-ounce) can chickpeas (garbanzo beans), rinsed and drained

2 tablespoons all-purpose flour

1 large egg white

½ teaspoon salt

¼ teaspoon red pepper

1 (10-ounce) package frozen chopped spinach, drained
and squeezed dry

¾ cup finely grated carrot

¼ cup minced green onion

4 (1½-ounce) hamburger buns

4 large romaine lettuce leaves

4 slices tomato

20 thin slices cucumber

4 thin onion slices

¼ cup Creamy Cucumber Ranch Salad Dressing (p. 212) (optional)

Combine bulgur and ⅔ cup boiling water in small bowl; let stand
30 minutes or until water is absorbed and bulgur is tender.

Meanwhile, in a small nonstick skillet, heat the olive oil over
medium heat; add the walnuts and sauté 3–4 minutes or until fragrant.
Stir in cumin; sauté 1 minute. Transfer to a large bowl.

Place the chickpeas, flour, egg white, salt, and red pepper in a food
processor, and process until smooth. Add this mixture to the walnuts in
large bowl. Add the plumped bulgur, spinach, carrot, and green onion;
mix well.

Shape into four ¾-inch-thick patties.

Grill or broil the burgers on a rack coated with vegetable cooking
spray, until browned and cooked, about 5 minutes per side.

Arrange the lettuce, tomato, cucumber, and onion slices on buns,
top with the burgers, and serve immediately. If desired, top each burger
with 1 tablespoon Creamy Cucumber Ranch Dressing, or 2 teaspoons
mustard or ketchup.

Yield: 4 servings.

Nutritional Information Per Serving. Calories: 445. Energy Density: 1.4.
Carbohydrate: 69 g. Fat: 13 g. Protein: 17 g. Fiber: 13 g. Sodium: 742 mg.
Good Source: Vitamin C, Fiber.

With Creamy Cucumber Ranch Dressing. Calories: 466.

With ketchup or mustard. Calories: 454.

Bean Cheese Burrito

This is great to make the night before and take to the office for lunch.

1 (12-inch) fat-free flour tortilla
⅓ cup drained, canned pinto or black beans, mashed
¼ cup commercial chunky salsa, divided
¼ cup (1 ounce) shredded reduced-fat (2 percent) Cheddar cheese
1 tablespoon sliced green onion
1 tablespoon sliced pitted ripe olives
2 tablespoons diced seeded tomato
½ cup lightly packed, thinly sliced romaine lettuce
2 tablespoons fat-free sour cream

Preheat the oven to 350 degrees F.

Tear off a 12-inch sheet of aluminum foil. Place the tortilla in the center of the foil. Stir together the beans with 2 tablespoons salsa. Spoon the bean mixture in a strip in the middle of the tortilla, but slightly off center. Leave a 1-inch border at each end. Top with cheese, green onion, olives, and tomato.

Fold in the short ends of the tortilla over the bean mixture; fold in the side of the tortilla closest to the bean mixture, and roll up tightly. Wrap in aluminum foil; can be cooked immediately or refrigerated up to 2 days. Bake for 10–15 minutes or until hot.

To serve, place the burrito on a serving plate and top with lettuce, the remaining 2 tablespoons salsa and sour cream.

Microwave directions: Follow the directions above, but use heavy-duty microwave-safe plastic wrap instead of aluminum foil. Microwave on high for 20 seconds, rotate 180 degrees, and turn over, and microwave an additional 20–30 seconds or until hot.

Yield: 1 serving.

Nutritional Information Per Serving. Calories: 350. Energy Density: 1.1. Carbohydrate: 49 g. Fat: 8 g. Protein: 18 g. Fiber: 16 g. Sodium: 1,149 mg. Good Source: Fiber.

Pasta Primavera

Combining pasta with fresh vegetables makes for a filling, low-calorie dish.

2 cups bow tie pasta, uncooked

1 cup small broccoli florets

½ cup sliced carrot

½ cup sliced celery

½ cup red bell pepper (½ medium), cut into thin 2-inch-long slices

½ cup cut fresh green beans

¼ teaspoon salt

¼ teaspoon freshly ground pepper

1 cup cherry tomatoes, halved

¼ cup (1 ounce) freshly grated Parmesan or Asiago cheese

2 tablespoons minced fresh basil (or fresh parsley)

2 tablespoons extra-virgin olive oil

Cook the pasta in 3 quarts boiling, salted water in a large saucepan according to package directions. During the last 3 minutes of pasta cooking time, add the broccoli, carrots, celery, bell pepper, and green beans to the saucepan.

Drain the pasta and vegetables well in a colander, and transfer immediately to a large serving bowl. Sprinkle with salt and pepper, and toss. Add the tomatoes, cheese, and basil, drizzle the olive oil, and toss well.

Serve immediately, or store in a covered container in the refrigerator, and serve as a cold pasta salad. To reheat after refrigeration: For each 1½-cup serving, cover and heat in the microwave on high for 60–90 seconds or until hot, stirring once.

Yield: 4 servings of 1½ cups each.

Nutritional Information Per Serving. Calories: 260. Energy Density: 1.3. Carbohydrate: 32 g. Fat: 11 g. Protein: 9 g. Fiber: 3 g. Sodium: 291 mg. Good Source: Vitamin A, Vitamin C.

Apple Crumble

A *Volumetric* apple brown Betty.

6 cups peeled, thinly sliced Granny Smith apples (about 4 large)

¾ cup firmly packed light brown sugar, divided

2 tablespoons water

3 tablespoon thawed frozen apple juice concentrate, divided

2 teaspoons cornstarch

¾ teaspoon ground cinnamon

⅔ cup regular oats, lightly toasted*

½ cup All Bran with Extra Fiber cereal

¼ cup whole-wheat flour

¼ cup all-purpose flour

1 teaspoon ground cinnamon

2 tablespoons canola oil

Preheat the oven to 400 degrees F.

Combine the apples, ¼ cup brown sugar, water, 1 tablespoon apple juice concentrate, cornstarch, and ¾ teaspoon cinnamon in a large bowl, and toss well to coat the apples. Spoon the mixture into a shallow, 1½-quart baking dish coated with cooking spray.

Combine the oats, flour, and 1 teaspoon cinnamon, the remaining ½ cup brown sugar, the remaining 2 tablespoons apple juice concentrate, and the canola oil in a food processor, and pulse until it is just blended. Sprinkle over the apple mixture.

Cover with aluminum foil and bake for 25 minutes.

Uncover and bake for 15 minutes or until the fruit is tender and the topping is crisp. Serve warm or at room temperature.

*Preheat the oven to 400 degrees F., spread oatmeal on the baking pan, and bake for 5–8 minutes.

Yield: 6 servings of ¾ cup each.

Nutritional Information Per Serving. Calories: 245. Energy Density: 1.8.
Carbohydrate: 51 g. Fat: 6 g. Protein: 3 g. Fiber: 7 g. Sodium: 36 mg.
Good Source: Fiber.

Red, White, and Blue Trifle

This is a colorful, layered dessert.

1 (15-ounce) carton fat-free ricotta cheese

1 (8-ounce) carton fat-free or low-fat lemon or vanilla yogurt

½ cup powdered sugar

2 teaspoons vanilla extract

1 (10-inch) round commercial angel food cake, cut into 1-inch cubes

1 medium banana

2 teaspoons lemon juice

2 cups frozen, thawed raspberries

2 cups fresh blueberries

2 cups sliced strawberries

1½ cups frozen fat-free whipped topping, thawed

Combine the ricotta, yogurt, powdered sugar, and vanilla in an electric blender, and process until smooth. Set aside.

Layer one-third of the cake cubes in the bottom of a large trifle bowl or deep serving bowl. Spoon one-third of the ricotta mixture evenly over the cake cubes.

Peel and slice the banana, and toss the slices with lemon juice.

Layer one-third of the banana, raspberries, and blueberries on top. Repeat with layers of cake, ricotta mixture, and fruit twice. Spread the whipped topping over the top layer of fruit. Cover and refrigerate at least 2 hours before serving.

Yield: 15 servings of 1 cup each.

Nutritional Information Per Serving. Calories: 205. Energy Density: 1.2.
Carbohydrate: 40 g. Fat: 1 g. Protein: 8 g. Fiber: 2 g. Sodium: 284 mg.

Brownie Sundae Soufflés

¼ cup Hershey's chocolate syrup

4 teaspoons finely chopped pecans or peanuts

½ cup powdered sugar

¼ cup unsweetened Dutch process cocoa

1 tablespoon all-purpose flour

½ cup low-fat (1 percent) milk

1 large egg yolk

½ teaspoon vanilla extract

2 large egg whites, at room temperature

⅛ teaspoon cream of tartar

2 tablespoons sugar

Preheat the oven to 350 degrees F.

Coat four 4- to 5-ounce soufflé cups with vegetable cooking spray.

Spoon 1 tablespoon chocolate syrup in the bottom of each soufflé cup. Spoon 1 teaspoon nuts on top of the syrup.

Combine the sugar, cocoa, and flour, and sift into a medium saucepan. Whisk in the milk until smooth. Cook over medium-low heat for about 10 minutes or until thickened, stirring constantly. Remove the saucepan from the heat.

Beat the egg yolk and vanilla in a small bowl, and whisk in one-fourth of the cocoa-milk mixture from the saucepan. Whisk the egg yolk mixture into the remaining cocoa-milk mixture in the saucepan. Set aside.

Beat the egg whites and cream of tartar in a small mixing bowl until soft peaks form. Gradually sprinkle in 2 tablespoons sugar, beating until stiff peaks form.

Fold about one-fourth of the egg whites into the cocoa-milk mixture in the saucepan, and then fold cocoa-milk mixture into the remaining egg whites in the mixing bowl. Spoon this soufflé mixture evenly in soufflé cups. (Soufflés may be cooled, covered, and refrigerated for up to 1 day before cooking.)

Place the soufflé cups on a baking sheet, and bake 15–17 minutes, or until the soufflés are puffed and set.(If you are using refrigerated soufflé mixture prepared in advance, bake for about 24 minutes.)

Serve immediately.

Yield: 4 servings.

Nutritional Information Per Serving. Calories: 200. Energy Density: 2.2. Carbohydrate: 37 g. Fat: 4 g. Protein: 5 g. Fiber: 2 g. Sodium: 54 mg.

Carrot Spice Cupcakes with Cream Cheese Frosting

1 (8-ounce) can crushed pineapple in unsweetened juice, undrained

1½ cups sifted cake flour

1 teaspoon baking powder

¼ teaspoon baking soda

¼ teaspoon salt

¾ teaspoon ground cinnamon

¼ teaspoon ground nutmeg

1 large egg

1 large egg white

⅓ cup low-fat or fat-free buttermilk

¼ cup canola oil

1 teaspoon vanilla extract

¾ cup sugar

1½ cups finely grated carrot

Cream Cheese Frosting (recipe follows)

Preheat the oven to 350 degrees F.

Drain pineapple in a wire mesh sieve, and press down on the pineapple to extract excess liquid. Reserve the juice separately for the frosting.

Sift the cake flour, baking powder, soda, salt, cinnamon, and nutmeg into a large bowl.

Combine the egg, egg whites, buttermilk, oil, and vanilla, and whisk until smooth. Whisk in the sugar.

Add the egg-buttermilk mixture to the flour in the bowl, and whisk until the dry ingredients are moistened. Fold in the carrot and reserved pineapple.

Spoon the batter evenly into paper-lined muffin pans. Bake 15–20 minutes or until a wooden pick inserted in center comes out clean. Let the cupcakes cool in the pans for 10 minutes, and then remove them from the pans and cool completely on wire racks.

Spread 1 tablespoon pineapple Cream Cheese Frosting on each cupcake.

Yield: 12 cupcakes.

Note: After cupcakes are cooled, they may be sealed in heavy-duty, reclosable plastic bags and frozen up to 1 month. Refrigerate the Cream Cheese Frosting. To serve, thaw the desired number of individual cupcakes, let 1 tablespoon frosting for each cupcake soften, and frost.

Cream Cheese Frosting

2 ounces (¼ cup) cold reduced-fat block cream cheese

1¾ cups powdered sugar, divided

1 tablespoon reserved pineapple juice

1 teaspoon vanilla extract

Place the cream cheese in a medium bowl. Sift 1 cup of the sugar over the cream cheese with a fine wire mesh sieve, and work the sugar into cream cheese with a spatula. Stir in the pineapple juice and vanilla, and work in the remaining sugar until spreadable and smooth.

Yield: 12 servings of 1 tablespoon each (about ¾ cup).

Nutritional Information Per Cupcake with Frosting. Calories: 220. Energy Density: 1.7. Carbohydrate: 39 g. Fat: 6 g. Protein: 3 g. Fiber: 1 g. Sodium: 139 mg.

Oat Bran Crepes with Ginger Peach Compote

5 tablespoons all-purpose flour

¼ cup oat bran

2 tablespoons sugar

1 large egg

½ cup evaporated fat-free milk

⅓ cup water

2 teaspoons canola oil

1 teaspoon vanilla extract

¼ teaspoon salt

Vegetable cooking spray

Ginger Peach Compote (recipe follows)

2 tablespoons sliced almonds, toasted

2 tablespoons powdered sugar

Combine the flour, oat bran, and sugar in a blender, and process until the oat bran is finely ground. Add the egg, milk, water, canola oil, vanilla extract, and salt, process until smooth. Cover and refrigerate the batter for 1 hour.

Preheat the oven to 375 degrees F.

Spread the almonds on a baking sheet, and bake for 5–7 minutes, until lightly toasted. Set aside.

Remove the crepe batter from the refrigerator. Coat an 8-inch non-stick skillet or seasoned crepe pan with cooking spray, and heat over medium-high heat until a drop of water dances on the surface. Ladle 3 tablespoons crepe batter all at once into pan, and swirl to coat the bottom evenly.

Cook for 30–45 seconds or until the crepe is lightly browned on the bottom. Loosen the crepe with a spatula, flip it over, and cook for 20–30 more seconds or until the bottom is lightly browned. Transfer the crepe to a plate, and cover it with wax paper. Repeat with the remaining batter, stacking the crepes between sheets of wax paper as they are cooked. There should be enough batter to make 6 crepes.

Coat an 11-inch x 7-inch x 2-inch baking pan with vegetable cooking spray. Spoon a heaping ¼ cup Ginger Peach Compote in a strip in the center of each crepe. Roll up each crepe and arrange crepes in the baking dish.

Bake, uncovered, 10–15 minutes or until hot. Sprinkle ½ teaspoon sliced almonds and sift 1 teaspoon powdered sugar over each crepe.

Yield: 6 servings.

Ginger Peach Compote

1 tablespoon cornstarch

1 tablespoon sugar

2 tablespoons Amaretto liqueur

1 tablespoon honey

1 tablespoon water

3 cups diced, peeled fresh or frozen peaches

2 tablespoons finely minced crystallized ginger

Combine the first five ingredients in a medium saucepan, and stir until the cornstarch dissolves. Add the peaches and ginger, and cook over medium heat for 15–20 minutes or until the mixture is hot and thickened, stirring frequently.

Yield: 6 fillings of ¼ cup each (about 1½ cups total).

Nutritional Information for Crepe with Compote. Calories: 219. Energy Density: 2.6. Carbohydrate: 43 g. Fat: 4 g. Protein: 6 g. Fiber: 5 g. Sodium: 153 mg.

Fudge Cake Brownies

2 ounces unsweetened chocolate, chopped

2 tablespoons canola oil

¾ cup All-Bran cereal

½ cup low-fat or fat-free buttermilk

4 large egg whites

2 teaspoons vanilla extract

1 cup grated zucchini

⅓ cup unsweetened cocoa powder

1 cup sugar

¼ cup all-purpose flour

½ teaspoon baking soda

¼ teaspoon salt

2 tablespoons powdered sugar

Preheat the oven to 350 degrees F.

Combine the chocolate and canola oil in a glass bowl, and cook in the microwave on high for 1½ to 2 minutes; stir until smooth. Let cool.

Pour the cereal into a food processor fitted with a knife blade, add the buttermilk, and pulse until the cereal is finely ground. Scrape down side of food processor, and let the mixture stand for 15 minutes.

Add the egg whites, vanilla extract, and zucchini, and pulse until just blended.

Pour the cocoa into a wire mesh sieve, and sift over a large bowl to remove lumps. Add the sugar, flour, baking soda, and salt, and stir with a wire whisk until blended. Stir in the cereal mixture. Pour into a 9-inch square baking pan coated with vegetable cooking spray.

Bake 30–33 minutes or until a wooden pick inserted in center comes out with a few moist crumbs attached. Cool before cutting. Sift powdered sugar over the top. Cut into 9 bars.

Yield: 9 servings.

Nutritional Information Per Serving. Calories: 205. Energy Density: 2.6. Carbohydrate: 34 g. Fat: 7 g. Protein: 5 g. Fiber: 4 g. Sodium: 88 mg.

Lemon Cheesecake Soufflé

9 vanilla wafer cookies, crushed

15 ounce part-skim ricotta cheese

1 8-ounce carton low-fat lemon yogurt

⅓ cup sugar

¼ cup fresh lemon juice

3 tablespoons all-purpose flour

1 egg yolk

2 teaspoons grated lemon rind

1 teaspoon vanilla extract

¼ teaspoon salt

5 large egg whites

⅛ teaspoon cream of tartar

¼ cup sugar

2 cups sliced strawberries, fresh blueberries, or fresh raspberries,
  or any combination

Preheat the oven to 350 degrees F.

Coat a 2-quart soufflé dish with vegetable cooking spray. Fold a
sheet of aluminum foil or parchment paper in half lengthwise, wrap it
around the outside of the soufflé dish, and secure it in plate with
kitchen string, so that it forms a collar that rises 3 inches above the
sides of the soufflé dish. Coat the inside of the soufflé dish with the
cookie crumbs, leaving any loose crumbs in the bottom of the dish.

Combine the ricotta, yogurt, ⅓ cup sugar, lemon juice, flour, egg
yolk, lemon rind, vanilla, and salt in a blender container, cover, and
process until the ricotta is smooth, scraping the sides of the blender as
necessary. Transfer the mixture to a large bowl.

Beat the egg whites and cream of tartar in clean large mixing bowl
at high speed of electric mixer until soft peaks form, and gradually add
the remaining ¼ cup sugar, beating until stiff peaks form.

Fold about one-fourth of the egg whites into the ricotta mixture,
and fold the ricotta mixture into remaining egg whites. Pour into the
prepared soufflé dish, and bake for 45 minutes or until the top is
golden and the center is set. Immediately spoon the soufflé into bowls,
and surround each serving with ¼ cup sliced berries.

Yield: 8 servings.

Nutritional Information Per Serving. Calories: 220. Energy Density: 1.5.
Carbohydrate: 30 g. Fat: 6 g. Protein: 11 g. Fiber: 1 g. Sodium: 210 mg.
Good Source: Vitamin C, Calcium.

Baked Pumpkin Custard

1 (15-ounce) can unseasoned pumpkin

1 (14-ounce) can fat-free sweetened condensed milk

1 cup egg substitute

⅓ cup water

2 teaspoons pumpkin pie spice

1½ teaspoon vanilla extract

⅛ teaspoon salt

Preheat the oven to 350 degrees F.

Beat all the ingredients in a large bowl with an electric mixer set at medium speed until the mixture is smooth.

Pour the mixture into an 8-inch round cake pan coated with vegetable cooking spray, cover the cake pan with aluminum foil, and place it in a larger baking pan. Pour hot water into the larger baking pan to a depth of 1 inch.

Bake for 1¼ hours or until a knife inserted in center comes out clean. Remove the pan from water, uncover, and let cool on a wire rack at least 30 minutes.

Serve at room temperature or cover and refrigerate overnight. Loosen the edges with a knife, and invert the custard onto a serving plate.

Yield: 8 servings.

Nutritional Information Per Serving. Calories: 190. Energy Density: 1.4.
Carbohydrate: 35 g. Fat: 1 g. Protein: 8 g. Fiber: 2 g. Sodium: 133 mg.
Good Source: Vitamin A.

Strawberry Banana Smoothie

Keep sliced fruit in your freezer, so you can make one of these at a moment's notice!

1 medium banana
1½ cups sliced fresh strawberries
2 cups ice cubes
½ cup water
½ cup low-fat (1 percent) milk
1 (8-ounce) carton fat-free, sugar-free strawberry yogurt*
1 tablespoon honey
1 teaspoon vanilla extract

Peel and slice the banana; you should have about 1½ cups. Arrange the banana and strawberry slices on a baking sheet, and freeze until solid. Use immediately, or transfer to a heavy-duty, reclosable plastic bag, and store in the freezer up to 2 weeks.

Place ice cubes in a heavy-duty, reclosable plastic bag, and crush with a rolling pin.

Put 1 cup crushed ice in a blender container, and the water, milk, yogurt, honey, vanilla, and frozen fruit. Cover and process until smooth.

Yield: 2 servings of 2 cups each.

*Regular fat-free yogurt is fine, too, but adds 55 more calories per serving.

Nutritional Information Per Serving. Calories: 215. Energy Density: 0.5. Carbohydrate: 44 g. Fat: 1 g. Protein: 7 g. Fiber: 4 g. Sodium: 88 mg. Good Source: Vitamin C.

Pineapple Peach Smoothie

1 cup cubed pineapple, canned or fresh

1½ cups chopped frozen unsweetened peaches

2 cups ice cubes

1 cup water

1 (8-ounce) carton fat-free, sugar-free peach yogurt*

1 tablespoon honey (optional)

1 teaspoon vanilla extract

Arrange the pineapple cubes on a baking sheet, and freeze until solid. Use immediately, or transfer to a heavy-duty, reclosable plastic bag, and store in the freezer up to 2 weeks.

Place ice cubes in a heavy-duty, reclosable plastic bag, and crush with a rolling pin.

Place 1 cup crushed ice in a blender container, and add the water, milk, yogurt, vanilla, and frozen fruit. Cover and process until smooth. Taste, and if needed, add the honey, cover, and process again.

Yield: 2 servings of 2 cups each.

*Regular fat-free yogurt is fine, too, but adds 55 more calories per serving.

Nutritional Information Per Serving. Calories: 215. Energy Density: 0.3. Carbohydrate: 49 g. Fat: 1 g. Protein: 5 g. Fiber: 6 g. Sodium: 58 mg.

Blue Moon Slushie

½ cup frozen blueberries

½ cup frozen blackberries

¼ cup grape juice

4 ice cubes

½ cup club soda, chilled

Combine the blueberries, blackberries, and grape juice in a blender container, and process until smooth.

Put the ice cubes in a heavy-duty, reclosable plastic bag, and coarsely crush with rolling pin. Add ½ cup coarsely crushed ice cubes to the blender container; process until slushy.

Pour the slushie into a tall glass, and stir in the club soda. Serve immediately.

Yield: 1 serving.

Nutritional Information Per Serving. Calories: 125. Energy Density: 0.3. Carbohydrate: 31 g. Fat: 1 g. Protein: 2 g. Fiber: 6 g. Sodium: 32 mg. Good Source: Fiber.

BREAKFAST

Double Bran Muffins

That monster muffin you grab on the way to work can top 500 calories. Instead, make these moist, fiber-rich ones. Freeze a bunch and toss one in the microwave for breakfast.

2 large eggs

¼ cup firmly packed light brown sugar

¾ cup fat-free buttermilk

⅓ cup applesauce

2 tablespoons vegetable oil

1½ cups wheat bran cereal, uncooked*

½ cup oat bran

½ cup all-purpose flour

1½ teaspoons baking powder

½ teaspoon baking soda

¼ teaspoon salt

Preheat the oven to 375 degrees F. Coat 9 muffin cups with vegetable cooking spray, or line them with foil or paper baking cups.

Beat the eggs and brown sugar in a medium bowl until smooth. Whisk in the buttermilk, applesauce, and oil. Stir in wheat bran cereal. Let the mixture stand at least 15 minutes and up to 30 minutes.

Combine the oat bran and remaining ingredients in a large bowl. Make a well in the center. Pour in the soaked bran mixture. Fold together with a rubber spatula just until dry ingredients are moistened.

Spoon the batter into muffin cups, filling ⅔ full. Bake 18–19 minutes or until a wooden pick inserted in centers comes out with a few moist crumbs attached. Remove from muffin cups, and serve warm, or cool on a wire rack.

Muffins may be frozen up to 2 weeks; after cooling completely, store them in a heavy-duty reclosable plastic bag in the freezer. To reheat, remove individual muffins from zip-top bag, and wrap each in a paper towel. Place in the microwave; microwave at medium-low power for 1–1½ minutes or until thawed and warm.

Yield: 9 muffins:

*This is not ready-to-eat, but hot cereal known as miller's bran.

Nutritional Information Per Muffin. Calories: 140. Energy Density: 2.5. Carbohydrate: 22 g. Fat: 5 g. Protein: 4 g. Fiber: 2 g. Sodium: 290 mg.

Zucchini Spice Variation. Omit the applesauce and add 1 cup grated zucchini, ½ teaspoon ground cinnamon, and ½ teaspoon pumpkin pie spice to the flour mixture. **Yield:** 9 muffins. Calories: 140.

Blueberry Orange Variation. Reduce buttermilk to ½ cup and add ¼ cup orange juice. Add 1 tablespoon freshly grated orange rind to the flour mixture. Fold in 1 cup fresh or frozen (do not thaw or drain) blueberries after mixing the batter. **Yield:** 10 muffins. Calories: 140.

Vegetable Frittata

Serve this for breakfast, brunch, lunch, or dinner.

1 tablespoon olive oil

1½ cups sliced mushrooms

1 cup sliced zucchini

1 cup cooked medium barley, made according to package
directions but without salt

1 cup chopped red or green bell pepper

1 cup sliced green onion

4 large eggs plus 8 large egg whites (or 2 cups egg substitute)

1 ¼ cups part-skim ricotta cheese

½ teaspoon salt

½ teaspoon freshly ground pepper

1 (10-ounce) package frozen chopped spinach, thawed
and squeezed dry

1 medium tomato, seeded and thinly sliced

2 tablespoons salsa (optional)

2 tablespoons fat-free sour cream (optional)

Preheat the oven to 450 degrees F.

Pour the olive oil into a 9-inch oven-proof skillet or quiche dish.
Add the mushrooms and zucchini to the skillet. Bake for 5 minutes
in the preheated oven. Remove the skillet from the oven, and layer in
the barley, the red pepper, and the green onion over the mushroom-
zucchini mixture. Top with tomato slices. Reduce the oven temperature
to 400 degrees F.

Combine the eggs and egg white (or egg substitute), ricotta cheese,
salt, and pepper in a blender or food processor; process until smooth.
Transfer to a bowl, and stir in the spinach. Pour evenly over the vegetables in the skillet; press down lightly on vegetables to allow egg mixture to seep through layers.

Bake the frittata, uncovered, for 35 minutes or until puffed and set.
Let stand 5 minutes before cutting into wedges. If desired, top each
serving with 2 tablespoons salsa and 2 tablespoons fat-free sour cream.

Yield: 6 servings.

Nutritional Information Per Serving. Calories: 225. Energy Density: 1.1.
Carbohydrate: 17 g. Fat: 10 g. Protein: 19 g. Fiber: 3 g. Sodium: 424 mg.
Good Source: Protein, Vitamin C, and Vitamin A.

Note: If you make this dish with 8 whole eggs instead of egg substitutes
or egg/egg white mixture, it adds 30 calories per serving.

Huevos Rancheros

2 whole-wheat 99 percent fat-free tortillas (6-inch diameter)

1 egg plus 2 egg whites (or ½ cup egg substitute)

¼ cup chopped onion

¼ cup chopped green onions

2 tablespoons water

Salt and pepper

1 tablespoon reduced-fat Cheddar cheese

¼ cup salsa

Combine egg and egg whites (or egg substitute) with onion, green
onions, water, and salt and pepper to taste in a small bowl.

Cover tortillas with a damp paper towel and cook in the microwave
on high for 30 seconds.

Grease a skillet with cooking spray and place over high heat. Pour
egg mixture into skillet, and fold and stir with a spoon or spatula until
the eggs are firm, about 3–5 minutes.

Place the tortillas on a plate, put half of scrambled egg in each tortilla, and top with the cheese and salsa.

Yield: 1 serving.

Nutritional Information Per Serving. Calories: 280. Energy Density: 0.9.
Carbohydrate: 33 g. Fat: 7 g. Protein: 20 g. Fiber: 2 g. Sodium: 738 mg.
Good Source: Protein, Vitamin C.

Vegetable Omelet

½ cup chopped spinach

½ cup sliced mushrooms

1 egg and 2 egg whites (or ½ cup egg substitute)

2 tablespoons low-fat (1 percent) milk

½ cup chopped tomatoes

3 tablespoons part-skim mozzarella cheese

Precook spinach and mushrooms in a covered microwave-safe bowl in the microwave on high for 1 minute.

Combine egg and egg whites (or egg substitute) with milk. Pour into a skillet greased with cooking spray over high heat. As the omelet cooks, place the spinach, mushrooms, tomatoes, and mozzarella in the center. Fold the omelet in half and cook for another 30 seconds to 1 minute.

Yield: 1 serving.

Nutritional Information Per Serving. Calories: 210. Energy Density: 0.7. Carbohydrate: 9 g. Fat: 10 g. Protein: 22 g. Fiber: 2 g. Sodium: 308 mg. Good Source: Protein, Vitamin A, Vitamin C, Calcium

Modifying Favorite Recipes

How can you make your meals more *Volumetric*? There are a few basic ways:

- Reduce fat.
- Add water.
- Increase fiber.
- Add fruits and vegetables, which provide both water and fiber.

While the principles are simple, they are also versatile. Either *subtracting* fat or *adding* water-rich ingredients will lower the energy density of a dish. When you do both, the results are even better. In the following examples, we'll show you how to modify favorite recipes to lower their energy density.

1. The Sandwich

It's lunchtime, and you order a bologna and cheese sandwich at your local deli: 2 slices whole-wheat bread, 2 slices (2 ounces) beef bologna, 1 slice (1 ounce) mild cheddar cheese, 1 piece lettuce, 1 tablespoon regular mayonnaise. It weighs 7 ounces, almost half a pound. Unfortunately, it also delivers 625 calories.

Your goal is to create a sandwich that's bigger yet delivers fewer calories. The final sandwich winds up with only 450 calories. To keep your calories at that level with the original deli lunch, you could eat only about three-quarters of the 625-calorie sandwich (*figure A,* next page).

That's not very satisfying. But how can we get to our *Volumetric* sandwich? First, we'll cut fat. Then, we'll add water and fiber by increasing the vegetables. Let's start with the fat-reduction techniques:

Substitute reduced-fat mayo for regular full-fat mayo.
Savings: 50 calories.

Substitute reduced-fat cheddar cheese for full-fat cheddar.
Savings: 20 calories.

Substitute lean roast beef for high-fat bologna.
Savings: 117 calories.

The sandwich, which weighs the same, now has only 438 calories. Great. But what if you could eat a bigger sandwich? You can, by adding vegetables. Let's say you add 2 slices tomatoes, 2 rings of green pepper, and 1 tablespoon alfalfa sprouts. That's a mere 14 calories.

Now your sandwich has only 452 calories. Its energy density has gone down from 3.2 to 1.8. You get to eat a bigger sandwich for fewer calories *(figure B)*.

Or, for the same calories as the original deli sandwich, you can eat a bigger sandwich, plus 1¼ cups of vegetable soup, and an apple.

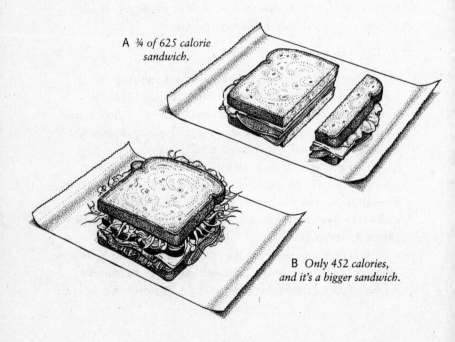

A ¾ *of 625 calorie sandwich.*

B *Only 452 calories, and it's a bigger sandwich.*

2. THE PIZZA

For dinner tonight, you make a quick pizza: a 10-ounce package of refrigerated pizza dough, dusted with 2 tablespoons cornmeal, to which you add 1 cup pasta sauce, 12 ounces shredded whole-milk mozzarella, a ¼ cup grated Parmesan cheese, and 24 slices pepperoni. That makes a pie that's 12 inches in diameter. You slice it up into 6 servings. Oops! Each slice has 450 calories. The energy density: 3.3.

We'll show you how to eat more pizza at only 290 calories a slice. If you wanted to take in that many calories with your pepperoni pizza, you'd be reduced to eating only 65 percent of a slice:

That won't do. So you make some changes.

First, you cut fat, both by choosing lower-fat foods and by using less cheese:

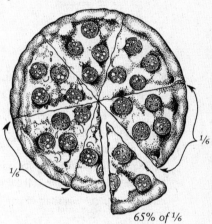

12" pizza in 6 equal parts

1/6

1/6

65% of 1/6

Substitute part-skim mozzarella for whole-milk mozzarella, and reduce the quantity from 12 ounces to 6 ounces. Savings per slice: 86.

Substitute a very lean Canadian bacon for high-fat pepperoni. Savings per slice: 84.

Now you've saved 170 calories, so a slice has only 280 calories. But is a single slice going to satisfy you for dinner? If not, make it *Volumetric*! How? To make the pizza chunkier, use diced fresh tomatoes (with basil, oregano, and garlic) instead of commercial pizza sauce; that also saves you 13 calories per slice. Now add more water- and fiber-rich vegetables: layer 1½ cups broccoli florets, 1 cup sliced cauliflower, 1 cup sliced red peppers, ½ cup mushrooms, ½ cup onions, and ½ cup yellow squash on your pizza. That adds only 26 calories per slice.

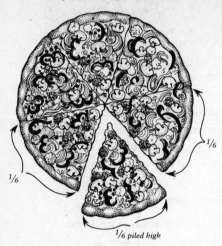

12" pizza in 6 equal parts

1/6

1/6

1/6 *piled high*

Now a slice has only 293 calories. The energy density has come down to 2.2. You are taking in fewer calories, and, with all those veggies, eating a lot more pizza.

Another way to put it: For the same calories as you get in the original pepperoni pizza, you can now eat 1½ slices of a slice that's much thicker.

3. THE MILKSHAKE

It's snack time. You'd like something that's under 100 calories. How about a milkshake? For 4 servings, you could mix together 1½ cups regular vanilla ice cream, ¾ cup reduced-fat (2 percent) milk, 2 cups strawberries, and 1 banana. The energy density is 0.9. Each 1-cup serving has about 180 calories. For 100 calories, you get less than ½ cup *(figure A)*.

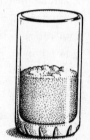

A ½ *cup of milkshake*

How can we make this more *Volumetric*? Let's replace the ice cream with the same amount of nonfat strawberry yogurt, and replace the milk with 1½ cups crushed ice, and keep the strawberries and banana. Instead of a milkshake, you've got a smoothie. Now its energy density is a mere 0.45. For 90 calories, you can enjoy a full cup *(figure B)*.

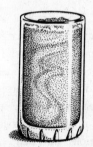

B *1 cup of a smoothie*

Part 6:

An Active Life

MANY OF YOU MAY FIND that losing the weight is easier than keeping it off. To maintain weight loss and prevent weight gain you need to increase physical activity. You don't have to become an athlete to keep weight off, but you do need to move your arms and legs every day, probably more than you are doing now. We'll show you the most effective ways of increasing physical activity for weight management.

The Exercise Prescription

EXERCISE ALONE IS OF MODEST HELP in weight loss. You simply can't burn that many extra calories a day. A brisk half-hour walk might burn 150 calories. Exercise-only weight loss plans often result in weight loss of a mere quarter-pound a week. Yet increased physical activity is critical for your weight management plan, and plays a key role in maintaining weight loss.

How can this be? The answer is simple: Weight loss is a different process from maintaining that weight loss. For weight loss, as we've shown, what matters is that you take in fewer calories than you burn. Diet-only plans result in an average weight loss of about 8 percent of body weight over 3–12 months: That's 16 pounds if you're now 200 pounds. Add exercise and you may take off a few more pounds. But physical activity will help keep the weight off.

THE ACTIVITY ADVANTAGE

One reason is metabolism. Reducing calories to lose weight causes you to lose not just body fat but also lean body mass, primarily muscle. Yet muscle is your metabolic ace in the hole. So you want to keep the proportion of muscle in your body high to facilitate weight loss maintenance. Even at rest, a pound of muscle burns many more calories than a pound of body fat. Lean body mass is the main determinant of the rate at which you burn calories at rest, so-called resting metabolic rate (RMR). Consider:

- Increasing physical activity slows the loss of lean body mass from weight loss and partly reverses the decline in RMR. If you lose weight by reducing intake, as much as 41 percent of the weight you lose will be lean body mass. But if you restrict calories *and* exercise, only 23 percent of your weight loss will be lean body mass.

- When you exercise, you not only burn calories but keep burning them at a higher rate for several hours later. People who are regularly physically active have a higher resting metabolic rate than people who are inactive.

- Exercise builds muscle. Resistance or weight training is particularly effective at building muscle, but any aerobic activity that works the long muscles of the legs and arms (walking, jogging, swimming, cross-country skiing) does so, too.

There's another reason that physical activity is indispensable to weight management: *It helps people make a commitment to a healthier lifestyle.* Regular physical activity is one of the most reliable ways to boost mood, lower anxiety, curb depression, improve sleep, and improve your sense of self-esteem. It makes you feel good, and that's been shown to help people stick with a weight loss program. "Exercise makes people feel better," says Cooper Institute's Steven Blair. "It also gives you a sense of self-efficacy, which makes it easier to maintain a good eating plan."

COUNTING CALORIES ON YOUR FEET

Calories count, whether you put them in your body as food, or burn them. "For weight management, the important thing is the total number of calories you burn," says University of Colorado medicine professor James O. Hill. "The real message is, 'Do something and do more of it.'"

To Burn 150 Calories

If you burn an extra 150 calories a day, you'll lose an extra pound a month, and make it easier to keep the weight off. Here's how:

- Wash and wax your car for 45–60 minutes.

- Play volleyball for 45 minutes.

- Garden for 30–45 minutes.

- Walk 1¾ miles in 35 minutes (3 miles/hour).

- Shoot basketball baskets for 30 minutes.

- Engage in social dancing for 30 minutes.

- Walk 2 miles in 30 minutes (4 miles/hour)

- Swim laps for 20 minutes.

- Play a basketball game for 15–20 minutes.

- Bicycle 4 miles in 15 minutes.

- Run 1½ miles in 15 minutes.

- Shovel snow for 15 minutes.

- Walk up and down stairs for 15 minutes.

Source: National Institutes of Health.

People who have lost a substantial amount of weight, and kept it off, often engage in physical activity like brisk walking for an hour or even more each day, well beyond the daily 30 minutes that's recommended for general health. "We're giving people a false sense that 30 minutes is all that you need," says Hill. Says Blair, "If you've lost weight, strive for at least 45 minutes a day. An hour would be better."

You needn't spend an hour at the gym each day. When you read the word *exercise*, you may envision Spandex-clad runners speeding by on the local track. You needn't become an athlete. You just have to move, frequently. "At the end of the day, it's the total calories you've spent that matters," says Blair.

Nor do you need to get all your activity at one time. If you start a walking program, you can go for 20 minutes three times a day, or even 10 minutes six times a day. "Accumulating" minutes of physical activity is beneficial for both weight management and health promotion.

Another effective approach is to become more active in ways that don't *feel* like exercise. Simply increasing "lifestyle activity" is a remarkably effective weight loss tool, according to weight management researchers at Johns Hopkins University in Baltimore. When overweight women lost weight on their program, some were instructed to engage in a structured aerobics exercise class as part of the maintenance phase. But another group was simply shown how

Should You See a Doctor First?

If you are currently inactive, you may want to talk with your doctor before beginning a new exercise program. You should definitely see a doctor first if you answer yes to any of the following questions:

- Has a doctor ever said you have heart problems?

- Do you frequently suffer from chest pains?

- Do you often feel faint or have dizzy spells?

- Has a doctor ever said you have high blood pressure?

- Has a doctor ever told you that you have a bone or joint problem, such as arthritis, that has been or could be aggravated by exercise?

- Are you over the age of 65 and not accustomed to exercise?

- Are you taking prescription medications, such as those for high blood pressure?

- Is there a good medical reason, not mentioned here, that you should not exercise?

Source: British Columbia Department of Health, in *Physical Activity and Weight Control*, from National Institute of Diabetes and Digestive and Kidney Diseases, National Institutes of Health.

to increase the physical activity in their daily lives: Walk more each day, perform more yard work and household chores, use the stairs more often, and so on. Both groups lost weight, but after a year, the lifestyle exercise group also kept virtually all the weight off, while the aerobic exercisers regained several pounds. Why? More of the lifestyle exercisers were very physically active a year later.

So make it a goal not only to engage in more intentional exercise like a walking program but to reduce your "sedentary time." Turn off the television set; the more you watch, the heavier you'll be, statistics tell us. Get off public transportation one stop early and walk the rest of the way, park farther from work or shopping, do errands on foot or on a bicycle rather than always jumping in the car, start a garden, walk up stairs, develop an active hobby, get a manual lawnmower, take your kids for a walk, walk your dog more often.

BURNING CALORIES

Your goal for weight management should be to increase the total number of calories you burn each day. Do it gradually, especially if you've been quite sedentary. Try walking for 10 minutes one day, and increase your walk by a few minutes each day. Once you've attained a reasonable level of fitness, you may wish to try these additional approaches to improve the effectiveness of your program:

- *Duration*. Physical activity that lasts longer than 45 minutes burns fat more efficiently. If you're walking, aim for a walk of an hour or longer at least once a week.

- *Intensity*. While most of your physical activity should be of moderate intensity, incorporating some higher-intensity workouts into your program can be helpful, recent research finds. Moderate intensity is defined as 50–70 percent of your maximal heart rate, while high intensity is 70–85 percent. To determine the intensity of your exercise, subtract your age from 220; that's your maximal heart rate in beats per minute. (If you are obese, with a BMI over 30, subtract your age from 200.) Let's say your maximal heart rate is 180. To exercise at

75 percent intensity, you'll multiply your maximal heart rate by 0.75. This gives you your target level of 135 heartbeats per minute. You can stop to take your pulse while exercising to compare it to this target.

- *Resistance.* A resistance or strength-training program, either with weights or machines, is an excellent part of a weight management program. It builds muscle, which boosts metabolic rate. You don't need to join a gym: A weight-lifting program at home with dumbbells is sufficient. Resistance "rubber bands" are another inexpensive option.

BUT WON'T EXERCISE JUST MAKE ME HUNGRY?

Many people fear that increasing exercise will simply stimulate the appetite, so they will make up the calories they burn by eating more. It's an unfounded fear. In fact, the human body may need some physical activity for satiety and hunger regulatory systems to work properly. There is some evidence, especially in overweight people, that increasing physical activity also helps prevent overeating that's not based on hunger. One thing is clear:

If you exercise more, you won't make up those calories during that day or the next. This has been shown repeatedly. In one study, even two intense exercise bouts a day didn't affect how much the subjects ate. "In the short term, you don't make up for all the calories you burn in exercise," says Jim Hill. "There's no increase in the number of calories people consume."

In the long term, endurance athletes do consume extra calories. But the caloric deficit created by increasing exercise can go on for a long time. Endurance swimmers, who burn up between 500 and 3,500 calories a day in exercise, for example, have been shown to stay in a caloric deficit for as long as 55 days. Contrast this to skipping even one meal: You'll feel hungrier at the next meal. So walk 2 miles before dinner. You'll not only burn 150 calories, you won't feel like eating more.

How to Walk

Walking is the best weight management physical activity for many people. It's practically injury-free. It's easy to fit into a busy lifestyle. Here's how:

- **Start gradually.** If you are overweight and sedentary, build up walking endurance with a 10-minute walk at a comfortable pace. Do this three times this week. Next week, walk three times for 15 minutes each. Gradually, over several weeks, build up so you can walk for 45–60 minutes 5 days a week.

- **Stretch.** Do light stretching before your walk, and then a longer stretch after your walk, when your muscles are warmed up.

- **Warm up.** Start slowly and build up to your regular pace over 5 minutes.

- **Find your pace.** A brisk yet sustainable pace for most people is between 15 and 20 minutes to walk a mile.

- **Accumulate.** When you can't fit in a long walk, take several shorter walks. You'll burn as many calories. Try a 15-minute walk before lunch each day.

- **Include longer walks.** Longer walks are particularly effective for burning body fat. Try to fit in two or three walks of 45–60 minutes each week.

- **Vary the intensity.** If you're reasonably fit, throw in more challenging workouts. This is useful if you've been walking for months but have reached a weight plateau, or you start to regain. In a 45-minute walk, do 5 minutes at a faster clip. Each week, add more faster minutes until 20 minutes or so of each workout is really brisk.

- **Alternate hard/easy days.** After a long, hard workout, your body needs time to recover. If you put in a vigorous walking workout on Saturday, try a long, more comfortable walk on Sunday.

- **Try weights.** Once you can walk 45 minutes or more at 3–4 miles per hour, you can add hand or ankle weights (or both) to burn more calories. Swing your arms as you walk. (Skip weights if you have high blood pressure.)

- **Cool down.** Walk more slowly for the last 5 minutes, until your heartbeat returns to close to normal.

- **Drink water.** Drink 1 cup every 20 minutes while you're walking, plus another one when you stop.

- **Rest.** As you build up endurance, give your body time to replenish energy: Get enough sleep.

Where to walk? Anywhere you want, of course. But you may want to look into mall walking clubs, where individuals meet, often in the morning before the mall opens, to walk its measured lengths in groups. It's a safe environment, protected from inclement weather. Because it's done with a group, it combines the elements of social support that have been shown to help people stick with exercise and other lifestyle changes. To find a group, ask at your local mall.

THE LOOPHOLE

Becoming more active is the nearest thing in weight management to a magic bullet. It makes you healthier, increases your metabolic rate, makes it easier to keep weight off, improves your mood, and helps you stay committed to a sensible eating plan. Yet, like everything that involves human beings, you can undo many of these benefits if you play mind games. If you decide to "reward" yourself for your workout with a treat that you would otherwise skip, you'll easily make up for the calories burned. One survey of 3,000 fitness instructors in health clubs found that a common mistake in exercisers was the consumption of highly caloric sports drinks and "energy bars" after workouts. As Neil A. King of the University of Leeds in England writes, "One phenomenon that has recently been confirmed is that selecting high-fat (energy-dense) foods after exercise will completely reverse the negative energy balance created by exercise."

SUMMARY

- Increasing your physical activity is critical for maintaining weight loss and preventing weight gain.

- Exercise keeps your resting metabolic rate higher while you lose weight, primarily by preserving your body's lean body mass (muscle), which burns calories faster than does body fat, even at rest.

- Becoming more active helps you feel better and makes it easier to stick to a sensible eating plan.

- The most important goal is to increase the total calories that you burn each day.

- Start gradually, especially if you are sedentary, and build up over several weeks.

- Aim for 45 minutes to 1 hour or more a day of physical activity.

- Walking is the best weight management activity for many people.

- Increase lifestyle activity by walking more, gardening, climbing stairs, watching less television.

- If you're reasonably fit, you can increase the effectiveness of your program by including bouts of longer duration (at least 45 minutes) and greater intensity.

- Resistance training with weights or machines is another excellent addition to a weight management program.

- Exercise won't make you hungrier. When people burn calories in physical activity, they don't make up those calories at meals. But don't reward yourself with energy-dense treats after a workout.

Six Stretches

Whether you walk, swim, bicycle, play basketball, or garden, the following stretches will help prevent injury. They were developed in consultation with fitness writer Royce Flippin, author of *Fit Again: 90 Days to Lifetime Fitness for the Over-35 Male*. They are appropriate for men and women at any age.

- **Calf-Achilles.** With your hands on a wall or the back of a chair, stand with your feet a few inches apart. Step backward with your right foot, so your toes are behind your left foot's heel. Bend both knees slightly, with your feet flat on the floor, and your weight over the right foot. Lean forward and down until you feel a stretch down the back of your calf and heel. Hold for 15–30 seconds. Reverse position and repeat to stretch left calf.

- **Hamstring.** Lie on your back and bend your left leg, keeping your left foot flat on the floor. With your right leg straight (don't lock your knee), lift it from the hip until you feel a gentle stretch running down the back of your thigh. You may want to clasp your hands behind your knee to assist in the stretch, or place a towel just above the back of the knee. Hold for 15–30 seconds. Repeat with the other leg.

- **Lower back.** Lie on your back with your legs extended. Bend your right leg, and clasp your hands behind your right knee. Then pull your right knee toward your chest, keeping your left leg very straight. Hold it for 15–30 seconds. Repeat with your left leg, then with both legs together.

- **Hip flexor.** Kneel, with your left knee resting on the floor, and move your right leg forward so your right foot is flat on the ground and your right knee is directly over your right ankle. Gently lower your left hip, until you feel a stretching sensation in the front of your left hip. Hold for 15–30 seconds. Repeat with the position reversed.

- **Chest.** While you are standing or sitting, lace your fingers behind your back, so your palms are facing in toward your spine. Raise your hands slowly toward the ceiling, until you feel a stretching sensation in the front of your chest. Don't arch your back, and keep your neck in a relaxed position. Hold for 15–30 seconds.

- **Neck.** Sitting in a chair, shrug your shoulders and then relax them slowly. Do this several times. Now, inhale deeply, and slowly drop your chin towards your chest; exhale and return to the starting position. Do this several times. Finally, sit with your chin tucked in slightly and inhale deeply, turning your head to the left as far as it will comfortably go. Exhale and return to your starting position, then repeat the stretch to the right side, using the same breathing pattern. Do this several times, too.

Part 7:

The Satiety Lifestyle

FOOD CHOICE PLAYS A CENTRAL ROLE in satiety. But it's not just the foods you choose that determines how much you eat. It's also the eating environment.

Do you eat more at parties? When dining with friends? At restaurants where the plates come out groaning with delectables? Would you eat more if you opened a big bag of snacks instead of a little one? If you skip breakfast or lunch, does that mean you'll eat fewer calories for the day, or will you more than make up the calories by overeating at subsequent meals? And if you've eaten until you're full at a meal, why is there always room for dessert?

The eating environment also includes your psychological state. Can emotions stimulate overeating? What about dieting itself? How can you learn to recognize biological hunger and satiety, and stop eating when your body gives you the signal that you're full?

In this section, we'll tackle these questions and many more.

Are You Hungry?

A hungry stomach will not allow its owner to forget it, whatever his cares and sorrows.
—HOMER, *The Odyssey*, 800 B.C.

WHEN YOU WERE THREE, you ate when you were hungry and stopped eating when you were full. By the time you were five, environmental cues, such as the amount of food on your plate, began to affect how much you ate. Now that you are an adult, you've learned to eat for many reasons besides hunger, such as:

- It's lunchtime.

- A surprise office birthday party materializes.

- A friend invites you to an impromptu early dinner.

- You're watching television and reach for a snack.

- You know there is chocolate in the cupboard.

- You are bored.

- You've been dieting for a week and suddenly "need" a treat.

For *Volumetrics* to work for you, you'll need to get back in touch with what hunger—and its satisfaction—feels like. It's not enough to learn how to choose a more satiating, lower-calorie dietary pattern. Satisfying hunger is only half the battle. You need to listen to your body's satiety signals, and learn ways to avoid eating when you are not really hungry. To effectively manage your weight, you'll need not only to feel full, but to actually stop eating!

EMOTIONAL EATING

Each of us, at times, eats for reasons that are based on emotions, rather than on the body's hunger. Ask yourself how well these statements describe you:

- When I am worried I eat more.

- I eat when I am mad.

- When I do something well I give myself a treat.

- When I am sad I eat more.

- When I am happy I eat more.

- When I am bored I eat more.

- I eat between meals even when I am not hungry.

Each statement describes a situation in which something other than hunger stimulates eating. "We often mix up other feelings with hunger," says Baylor College of Medicine's John Foreyt. "You start feeling anger, and you feel hungry. Depression, anxiety, and tension may all be linked to eating." The first step toward separating such emotions from hunger is to learn to label them correctly. Are you hungry, or just bored? Tired? Anxious? Once you label the emotion correctly, look for a more appropriate way to cope with it. Says Evelyn Tribole, coauthor of *Intuitive Eating*, "Ask yourself, 'What do I need other than food to cope with this feeling right now?'" For example:

- If you're angry, reduce your stress indirectly (taking a walk, talking to a friend) or directly (talk to the person who is making you angry).

- If you're lonely, call a friend.

- If you're bored walking home from work, take a new route.

- If you're depressed, exercise or see a movie. If depression lasts for weeks, get professional help.

- If you're fatigued, get some sleep.

- If you're anxious, try relaxation techniques such as deep breathing, or take a yoga class.

In this book, we have not addressed the complex psychological relationship you may have with food, eating, and your weight. But we can recommend several books to help you identify emotional triggers to overeating and overcome them: the above-mentioned *Intuitive Eating*, which helps readers get beyond a "dieting mentality" and eat for hunger; *Thin for Life*, by Anne M. Fletcher, M.S., R.D., which documents strategies of people who have successfully lost weight and kept it off; *Emotional Eating*, by Edward Abramson, Ph.D., a practical self-help book by a behavioral psychologist with experience treating patients who eat for emotional reasons; and *Living Without Dieting*, by John P. Foreyt, Ph.D., and G. Ken Goodrick, Ph.D., which lays out a nondiet behavioral approach to healthy weight control. However, if you have persistent anger, anxiety, or depression with a cause you can't identify, or you have a problem with binge eating, you may need professional therapeutic help to work through personal issues *before* you attempt to change your eating pattern.

Ironically, conventional dieting can interfere with sensitivity to hunger and satiety signals, and increase emotional overeating. After all, most diets ask you to consciously restrict what and how much you eat, often ignoring your body's hunger cues. If you restrict your food choices too much, you set up a good food/bad food mentality, which can easily translate into a good me/bad me mentality. That is, when you're good, you're in control, but as soon as you "break your diet," you'll overeat.

"When dieters are calm and in control, they tend to eat less than nondieters," says University of Toronto professor Janet Polivy. "But if dieters are coaxed into a situation where they eat and break the 'diet,' there's a 'what the hell?' effect. They'll think, 'My diet is broken, I'll just eat everything I'm not allowed to eat.' They give in to psychological hunger, not real hunger." Says Baylor's John Foreyt, "We all need some restraint—none of us can eat everything we want all the time—but when you go on a rigid diet, there's a sense of deprivation, and you start thinking about forbidden foods. Such restraint is linked to binge eating—and to weight gain."

Volumetrics is designed to help you get off the dieting roller coaster. That's why we emphasize normal, satisfying portions, and moderate, sustainable caloric reduction. Keep that long-term perspective: If you overeat at any one meal or day, simply move on and eat sensibly at the next opportunity. Don't try to "make up" the calories by greatly cutting calories the next day. Such a dieting mentality can lead to cycle of undereating and overeating. Nor are there any forbidden foods. Says Tribole, "I'd much rather have a client enjoy a Belgian chocolate than eat a whole box of fat-free cookies that don't satisfy."

MINDFULNESS

You don't have to feel deprived, bored, anxious, depressed, or joyful to eat too much. You can just stop paying attention. Awareness—including memory—is a surprisingly significant influence on eating behavior. At the University of Pennsylvania, two men with severe amnesia were served a meal, and ate it; 10–30 minutes later, they were served a second meal, and ate that, too; 10–30 minutes later, they started on a *third* meal. Without the memory of eating, their hunger did not decline.

If we don't pay attention, if we mindlessly eat, we may be like those amnesiacs. When surveyed, only 20 percent of obese men and women said they started eating because they felt hungry. Only 39 percent stopped eating because "I felt I had eaten enough." Like the amnesiacs, they paid little attention to the actual need for food.

So stay tuned to what your body is telling you about hunger and satiety. Eat without distractions such as driving, watching television, reading, loud music. Savor your food. Pay attention to the pleasure you get from the first bite, and continue to pay attention as you become more full and as each bite becomes just a little less pleasurable. When you are ready to stop eating, leave the table and begin another activity. If you want to read, listen to the radio, or watch television, now is the time.

I ATE IT BECAUSE IT WAS THERE

When food surrounds us, when it's in front of our noses, we may be enticed into eating when we're not hungry. Seeing a display of food, catching a whiff of the aroma of cookies baking, and even being reminded of food through television commercials can increase your desire to eat. That's why restaurants often present diners with a luscious dessert tray as soon as the entree is finished. Your senses, rather than your sense, may lead you into ordering a rich dessert.

Rather than "out of sight, out of mind," the lesson is "in sight, in the mind, and maybe in the mouth, too." In a large hospital cafeteria study, for example, the lid was kept on an ice cream cooler, and only 3 percent of obese and 5 percent of normal-weight subjects selected ice cream. But when the lid was taken off the cooler, so people could see the ice cream and reach it more easily, the percentages rose: 17 percent of the obese and 16 percent of the lean people ate ice cream.

Fortunately, the principle also works with lower-energy-dense foods such as soup and fruits. Just stockpiling soup in the house can increase the frequency with which you eat soup, finds Brian Wansink of the University of Illinois at Champaign-Urbana. Even the position of fruit in your house makes a difference. Wansink asked people to put fruit in the refrigerator, in a bowl in the kitchen, or in a bowl in the dining room. "Having fruit in a bowl in the kitchen had a tremendous impact," he says. They ate less fruit when it was in the dining room, and the least when it was in the fridge. His conclusion? "Stock the house with healthier foods!"

Chocolate Cravings

A *craving* is simply a strong appetite for a particular food. In one study, 49 percent of all food cravings were for chocolate. Why? Is it an addiction? Although chocolate does contain psychoactive substances, the levels are quite low. Attempts to show that chocolate causes a true addiction have been futile. At the University of Pennsylvania, Paul Rozin found that chocolate cravers preferred a milk chocolate bar over a white chocolate confection, which contains none of the pharmacologically active ingredients in cocoa. But this was because they liked the sensory properties of the chocolate bar better, not because it contained addictive ingredients. Consuming the white chocolate along with a capsule containing the pharmacological equivalent of cocoa didn't increase their liking for it.

People don't crave chocolate for some druglike effect, but because of its sensory properties and its calories. Chocolate tastes very good, and it is energy dense, so you can take in a large number of calories quickly. Indeed, eating any good-tasting, energy-dense food when you are hungry can create a craving for that food. In the United States, after chocolate, the food most people crave is pizza, which is aromatic, gooey, fatty, salty, and energy-dense. Repeatedly associating any food with a reduction of hunger can increase our appetite for that food.

The ready accessibility of chocolate snacks does mean that we frequently eat chocolate when we are hungry—it is a convenient way to tame between-meal hunger pangs. But by eating chocolate as a snack, you may be continually reinforcing your craving for it. Try to break that cycle. Have chocolate at the end of a meal when you are not very hungry. You are less likely to overindulge at that time and you can savor and enjoy its delicious flavor.

CAN YOUR DINNER COMPANION MAKE YOU FAT?

Whom we eat our food with influences what we eat and how much. Some of this is due to modeling, following the example of someone who is eating a particular type of food. Children do this, especially if the model is a friend or someone they admire, such as a TV character—not necessarily their parents! Adults also are inclined to follow others when it comes to eating.

Men and women respond to some social situations differently when it comes to food intake. Eating with the opposite sex has little impact on a man's food intake. But when a woman eats with an attractive male she eats less than with one she finds less attractive. It is thought that this is because women are socialized to believe that eating a small amount in a dainty fashion—slowly and in small bites—is more feminine. Surveys show that many people do perceive eating small meals to be more feminine.

In other social situations, people eat more. We conducted a study in which we offered groups of four men or four women spaghetti, salad, and dessert for dinner. On another occasion, we gave them the same foods to eat by themselves. If the people did not know one another, it made little difference whether they were alone or together. But when we tested groups of friends, they ate around 50 percent more when they were in the group setting. Most of the extra calories came from the dessert.

In a friendly social setting, many factors encourage overeating. We don't offer alcohol in our lab studies, but we do know that a drink can lower the resolve to restrain overeating. Good conversation may prolong the meal and distract us from paying attention to how much we are eating. When everyone else orders dessert, it is hard to sit and just watch.

So you need a plan. Eating alone is not the answer. We need friends and family, and social support is an important part of a weight management program. Besides, if you eat alone, it's easy to overeat from boredom or loneliness. One solution is to ask your friends to join you at eating establishments where watching what you eat is easier, for example, at a restaurant where you can order soup and a salad rather than just a burger and fries or nothing. Another is simply to be aware of the likelihood that eating together makes it easy to overeat. If it's a dinner party at your home or someone else's, you may suggest that after the meal, everyone retires to another room or engages in another activity, like a walk. In a restaurant, make a decision not to eat the bread before your food comes, to eat only an appropriate portion of a main dish, and/or not to eat dessert. You can learn to consume fewer calories in social situations, and still enjoy your friends!

THE MIND PLAYS TRICKS

Can your *ideas* about a food affect how much you eat? Do people who choose low-fat or fat-free foods use them as an excuse to eat more? For many people, the answer is yes.

We gave women a mid-morning yogurt snack and later served them lunch, at which they could eat as much as they wanted. Some yogurts were high in fat, others low. They were accurately labeled for fat content. We didn't tell the women about calories, though. Each yogurt, whether it was high or low in fat, had exactly the same calories. Yet when women ate yogurt with a "low-fat" label, they ate more at lunch than when they had eaten a yogurt labeled "high-fat." They didn't eat less at dinner after having the bigger lunch, either. So over the whole day, the women who had eaten the low-fat yogurt consumed more calories. The low-fat label, in other words, was a license to overeat. The women assumed that low-fat meant low-calorie.

As we've shown in this chapter, there are many reasons besides hunger and satiety that people eat, and overeat. When you lower the energy density of a meal, you can eat a normal portion with fewer calories. But if you stuff yourself, in the belief that this is a "safe" food, you may still wind up taking in too many calories. Don't let your mind run away with your mouth!

WHAT IS HUNGER?

So far we've explored some of the many reasons that people eat other than hunger. But what *is* hunger? It refers to the sensations you feel when your body needs food. It is distinct from "appetite," which refers to your desire for a particular type of food. What does hunger feel like? In a recent study at the Monell Chemical Senses Center in Philadelphia, university students described the sensations they experience when hungry:

- Stomach growls, stomach aches. These were the most commonly reported hunger sensations.

- Weakness, headaches, pain, dizziness, anxiety, loss of concentration, crave foods, thought of food, mouth waters. Each of these was reported, but less frequently.

When asked to indicate where on the body they felt hungry, the stomach region won hands down. The head was a distant second, and a few people described more general body sensations. When respondents were actually deprived of food, the greater the deprivation, the larger the area around the abdomen that was involved.

Hunger is the way your body gets your attention so that it gets the fuel it needs. When you're hungry, you seek food. In our evolutionary past, hunting and foraging took time and effort, but these days getting food has become very easy. As you select your meal or snack and begin to eat it, an exquisite sequence of events takes place that eventually signals your brain that you are no longer hungry. You're satiated, or, as most people put it, full.

SATIETY

Let's say you're hungry, it's your usual mealtime, and you decide to eat. You'll either prepare the food yourself, or get someone else to prepare it. Either way, you'll need to decide how much food is appropriate to satisfy your hunger. You'll begin with your previous experience with this type of food. How satisfying has this food been in the past? How much do you need? If it's chili, should you give yourself a half-cup, a cup, or even a cup and a half? If you ordered a large serving from a restaurant last week, and left feeling bloated, you may decide that a small side order is going to be fine today. As soon as the food is on your plate, you begin to eat—with your eyes.

How big a portion is it? The bigger the portion, the bigger the effect on "satiety," which refers to how full and satisfied you feel after eating. What actually brings your meal to an end, however, is the reversal of the symptoms of hunger, a process that's called satiation.

Satiation, the end of hunger, is affected not merely by your previous experience with the food and the visual cues you get about its size, but by a sequence of events that occurs after you start eating. These include smelling, chewing, and tasting the food; even the act of swallowing is important. These sensory experiences are important in signaling your body that food is arriving and needs to be digested. They also play a role in satiety. When you first begin to eat, good-tasting food tastes very good indeed. But as you continue to eat, the same food grows gradually less pleasurable–you experience sensory-specific satiety (see "Variety," p. 281). That's your body telling you that it's starting to feel satiated.

In this book, we've given you many different tactics to enhance satiety on fewer calories. The most important one, of course, is choosing a dietary pattern that's low in energy density. The main reason is that it allows you to eat a normal portion of food, so that many different components of your body's satiety system are activated. That way you'll be able to feel those calming, comforting feelings of satiety several times a day. You'll feel hungry at times—it's appropriate to be hungry before a meal—but you'll never have to *stay* hungry.

GETTING IN TOUCH WITH SATIETY

How do *you* experience hunger? Pay close attention and also notice whether it changes over the course of the day. Most people have little hunger right after a meal, but if asked to rate their hunger over the rest of the day, it rises steeply before habitual mealtimes. This is a natural pattern. Most people don't wait for the hunger to become uncomfortable, but feeling a little hungry at the start of a meal is good. *Volumetrics* helps you to control hunger and to maintain your usual cyclic pattern of hunger and satiety while eating fewer calories.

What sensations do you associate with stopping eating? Some people think of satiety as simply a reversal of what caused hunger. To some extent this is true, but satiety is associated with not only a reversal of the growls and aches in the stomach. The stomach also feels full. Indeed, the way we assess satiety in our lab is by asking people how full they feel.

"Full" doesn't mean "bloated," however. A bloated sensation is actually uncomfortable, and can bring on nausea. If you eat an appropriate amount, satiety is accompanied by a feeling of well-being. Often when we are hungry, we get grumpy and irritable. Eating reverses those feelings, so people feel calm after a meal. It may take practice to recognize how little food you need to feel satiated. "It doesn't take much to get full," says New York University professor Marion Nestle, who recently lost weight by stopping eating when she was no longer hungry. "You can't teach it—people have to learn it themselves."

Here are some other tips for becoming more sensitive to satiety:

- At the beginning of a meal, ask yourself, "Am I hungry?" You may want to rate your hunger on a scale of 1 to 10, 1 being painfully ravenous and 10 being so full you couldn't eat another bite. As you eat, periodically pause and ask yourself again, "Am I still hungry?" If your rating has reached 5, it may be time to stop eating.

- Realize that hunger is easily satisfied. If you are a little hungry in the afternoon, sometimes 100 calories will do. An apple or a yogurt may be enough.

- If you're really out of touch with hunger and satiety, try a routine. Eat breakfast, lunch, and dinner on a regular schedule for 10 days. Chances are, you'll start to feel hungry before each meal.

- Don't feel bad if you eat when you are not hungry sometimes, or continue to eat when you're full. That's okay. Everyone does. If you overeat at one meal, eat sensibly at the next.

In the end, it all boils down to one piece of advice: Listen to your body. It's easy to ignore or override satiety signals. We all do at times. Sometimes you may even decide to do so. That's fine. But the more attuned to how satiated you are becoming as you eat a meal or snack, the easier it will be to eat just enough food for your body.

SUMMARY

- Satisfying hunger is only half the battle—you also have to stop eating when you're no longer hungry!

- If you eat in response to emotion (boredom, anxiety, depression, happiness), identify the emotion that is triggering eating—and then find an appropriate nonfood way to handle that feeling.

- Dieting—chronic food restriction—can lead to overeating. Even when you are trying to lose weight, eat normal portions, reduce calories only modestly so that you lose weight gradually, and enjoy your favorite energy-dense foods in modest portions.

- It's easy to overeat when you're not paying attention. Whenever you can, eat without the distractions of television, radio, or reading.

- Accessibility can increase the amount of a food we eat. Take advantage of this by making energy-dense foods less readily available and making foods of lower energy density easy to grab.

- Eating with friends can increase the amount we eat. Manage this by smart food choices during social meals, such as skipping dessert.

- The experiences of hunger and satiety are created by a sequence of biological signals that involve the eyes, nose, mouth, throat, stomach, liver, pancreas, and small and large intestines. Eating a normal volume of food is essential to maintaining these satiety signals.

- Improve your sensitivity to satiety signals by asking yourself before a meal, and periodically throughout it, "On a scale of 1 to 10, how hungry am I now?"

Variety

New meat begets a new appetite.

—ENGLISH PROVERB

HUMAN BEINGS LOVE CULINARY VARIETY. It stimulates us to eat more. Although I (Barbara) have studied this effect for nearly two decades—and how to use it to manage weight—it wasn't until I attended an extraordinary pasta party in Italy that I realized just how strong the pull of variety is on our behavior. I was attending a conference. The program stated simply, "'Spaghetti party' at the Castellon di Lanciano: Tour of the Castle, cocktails and 'Spaghettata' on the menu."

A bus transported us to a remote castle in the mountains outside of Camerino, just east of Perugia, in the Italian coastal province of the Marches.

And then: nothing.

We waited for hours, getting hungrier and hungrier. Rumors circulated that our chef was famous for pasta. Finally, we were seated, and menus were presented. The first course was pasta. So was the second. And the third, the fourth . . . in all, fourteen courses of pasta. Then dessert. Apparently, this was a kind of Italian joke, a culinary hilarity. We started with gusto. The food was delicious, the wine matched it perfectly, and the company of colleagues could not have been better. Everyone was in a mood to enjoy the finest feast Italy could offer.

Each wonderful course was quite varied, in the shape of the pasta, the type of sauce, the flavors. We had thin pasta, thick pasta, tubular pasta, shell-shaped pasta. We started with a simple spaghetti in an olive oil–lemon sauce, followed by pasta served with basil sauce, with tuna sauce, with beans, with cooked proscuitto, baked with cheese, with meat sauce, with sausage, with tomatoes, with sweet gorgonzola cheese. Each was exquisitely prepared, aromatic, mouth-watering. Yet by the middle of the meal all but the heartiest eaters had given up. Our host attempted to revive appetites by announcing that our next course was a special new pasta that all of Italy was clamoring to try! Still, no one wanted . . . pasta. People got up, socialized, sipped their wine, and walked around as the last six or seven pasta dishes were served. Were we simply sated? So full we just couldn't take another bite? Perhaps.

Then dessert arrived. Suddenly, everyone sat down, eagerly, and ate the *dolce*, thin chocolate wafers with seasonal fruit, *con gusto*. By the end of this chapter you'll understand why the pasta had lost its appeal, but there was still an appetite for dessert. You'll appreciate why feasts throughout history have featured a wide variety of delectable foods that differ in taste, texture, even shape, while religious fasting periods often emphasize only a few simple foods.

Learning to manage the variety effect will help you incorporate the lessons of this book into everyday life, when you are no longer trying to lose weight but simply eating a satisfying diet without regaining the weight you've lost.

EVERYONE LOVES VARIETY

All humans and many animals seek dietary variety. Many mammals and birds, for example, have a preferred food, but once they've been able to eat it for a few days, they'll readily switch to a normally less-preferred food. Infants are also responsive to variety. When a breast-feeding mother varies her diet, eating foods like garlic that flavor her milk, her infant will drink more milk than when she has a blander diet that does not affect the milk's taste.

More significantly, newly weaned infants don't just stick to their favorite foods. In classic studies in the 1920s, Clara Davis undertook the undoubtedly messy business of letting infants feed themselves from a wide variety of nutritious foods. Some of the foods were very peculiar—bone marrow, for example. But these children did not have preconceived notions about foods, so they sampled everything including the cutlery, plates, and so on. Although they sometimes went on eating jags where they mostly ate bananas or some other food, in the long run they spontaneously ate a well-balanced, varied diet. Davis speculated that there must be very basic mechanisms that govern food selection, even in infants.

We now believe that a mechanism called sensory-specific satiety explains why the children ate varied diets. You already know that satiety is what you mean when you say "I'm full"; you no longer feel hungry and you stop eating. But how does this feeling arrive? You don't just eat until your stomach is full and then stop. It's more subtle. As you eat, the pleasure you get from the food you're eating slowly declines. If you're hungry, the first bite of a food you like is intensely delicious. Slowly, as you finish your meal, you find the food less attractive, less pleasant.

But a new course may reawaken your appetite. That's sensory-specific satiety: You become "full" for one specific sensory experience—the taste of pasta, for example, or even chocolate (believe it or not)—but not others. That is why at my Italian feast the dessert brought everyone back to the table. We had eaten more than enough pasta, we did not want any more salty, savory foods, but wanted something with a fundamentally different taste—sweet.

SENSORY-SPECIFIC SATIETY

What happens during a meal of many different foods, or courses, is that we experience satiety for each food as we eat it. But we are still "hungry" for foods we haven't eaten yet, particularly those that have different tastes, aromas, shapes, textures, and other sensory properties. To continue enjoying a meal, you'll switch from one food as it declines in pleasantness to another food, which remains appealing. But if all the foods presented are quite similar, you can't do this. That's what happened to us in Italy. Even though each pasta course was as different as a fine chef could make it, it wasn't different enough. It was still . . . pasta. One might say we experienced "pasta-specific" satiety.

Sensory-specific satiety plays an important role in ensuring that we eat a balanced diet. By switching from food to food, we increase the chances that we will consume all the nutrients we need. That is one reason that nutritionists advise us to eat a variety of foods.

The changes in pleasantness of foods occur very rapidly—while we are still eating a meal. Taste is central. Sweet foods affect the pleasantness of other sweet foods, while salty tastes affect other salty ones. People in our studies who ate chocolate pudding were less interested in sweetened fruit yogurt, for instance, but they were happy to eat salty potato chips. Conversely, eating a salty food like sausage decreased the pleasantness of salty cheese and crackers, but sweet foods were still attractive. So it's not surprising that after fourteen pasta courses, we were happy to get a sweet. If we had been offered fourteen sweet courses, though, a salty pasta course would have been just lovely.

Our response to food odors also changes as we eat. To me (Barbara) the smell of fresh-brewed coffee in the morning is intoxicating, but after I've had 2 cups, it's decidedly unpleasant. Not only does our response to the smell of a food change as we eat, but just smelling or chewing food, which releases the odors, can affect how much we like it. Some weight loss plans have been based on this idea. They suggest that if you smell food odors when you are hungry, you will feel satisfied and lose weight. This strategy may temporarily help you to resist a particular food, but that is probably not going to be enough to get the weight off. Also, you would have to smell the food odor for at least several minutes—just a whiff of a food might make you want it more!

VARIETY ENCOURAGES EATING

Meal patterns in many cultures stress the importance of different sensory qualities of foods throughout a meal. Differences in each course in taste, temperature, texture, aroma, color, and shape continue to pique culinary interest throughout the meal. This encourages you to keep eating and enjoying your food.

I've always wanted to do a study on a cruise ship where the passengers are tempted by huge buffets at every meal for a week. Would they continue to overeat or would they tire of the variety and become more picky about their choices? I suspect that the vast variety of tasty high-calorie foods that is so readily available in restaurants, in salad bars, at all-you-can-eat buffets, in supermarkets, and in our homes is part of the reason that we as a nation are getting fatter.

We know from studies at the Eating Lab that the variety of foods offered in a meal can affect how much is eaten. The more variety, the less likely it is that sensory-specific satiety will curb your eating. For example, when we fed students four courses of very different foods, they ate 60 percent more than when they had just one of the foods. Even when people had sandwiches with four different fillings, they ate a third more than when they had their favorite filling in all the sandwiches. Just varying the shape of food, pasta again, can increase intake. People ate 15 percent more when offered three shapes of pasta than when they had only their favorite shape. If you habitually eat 15 percent more even at one meal a day, such as lunch at the office cafeteria where there is so much choice that you can keep switching foods, it could easily add up to several extra pounds a year.

MANAGE VARIETY

The first place to manage the variety effect is to fully chew your food, enjoying its flavor, texture, and aroma. This enhances your appreciation of flavor and aroma and can help satiate you for that food. Look for ways to give yourself flavor with fewer calories. For chocolate, for example, try low-fat hot chocolate, or chocolate-flavored hard candies that take a while to consume, or low-calorie frozen chocolate desserts. If you crave the flavor of real chocolate, indulge with a small portion, and savor every moment of the flavor.

Be particularly careful around buffets, whether it's a salad bar at lunch hour, a cocktail party, a wedding, or a dinner party. It's so easy to load your plate with lots of different foods, each of which can stimulate appetite in turn. Here's what I (Barbara) do: Usually there is a large bowl of salad greens early on in a buffet—I make my plate look full with these. Other undressed salad veggies can be added, with a *small* amount of regular dressing or some low-fat dressing. Then I'll take really small portions (just a taste, really) of a number of different foods. That way I'm getting my variety and lots of sensory satisfaction. The trick is to ensure that I feel that I have eaten a satisfying portion of food. To do this I load my plate with foods that really fill me up with few calories—they are low-energy-dense *Volumetric* foods.

When it comes to a sit-down meal, remember that the traditional structure of a multicourse meal encourages eating. If you go out to a restaurant, and you start with an alcoholic beverage while you eat the bread on the table, then eat the appetizer, followed by your large main course with side dishes, and then find that two or three people at the table are ordering desserts "just for a taste," you're creating a situation where it's exceedingly easy to overeat. So you need a plan.

The basic strategy is to balance high-calorie courses with lower-calorie ones. If you know the main course is going to be big, make sure your appetizer is a light one, like asparagus or a salad with a low-calorie dressing. Another good tip is to eat a low-calorie, filling snack before you go out, so you don't arrive hungry and gobble up 3 pieces of bread before the first course arrives.

The real payoff, though, arrives when you realize that you don't have to "fight" sensory-specific satiety. If you make the right food choices, you can enlist the variety effect as your ally in the war against weight gain.

MUST I EAT BORING FOODS TO LOSE WEIGHT?

No! One lesson you *shouldn't* draw from this research is that it's a good idea to reduce the variety in your diet to control weight. Dietary variety is healthy: Nutritional balance, after all, is almost certainly why animals and humans evolved a taste for variety in the

first place. The desire for dietary variety is so strong that trying to
cut back on the number of different foods you eat is not only nutri-
tiona... foolhardy, but it's also a decidedly uphill battle. The good
news is: ... don't have to do it. The Japanese and the French, who
have more v... diets than we do, are also thinner. Dietary monotony isn't good ... which, it isn't fun, and, in the end, it's not the
way that people wh... cessful at controlling their weight eat.

You wouldn't kno... look at many diet books. Some
authors encourage curbing ... by having, for example, the
same lunch with the same few ... same time every day.
Many popular diets actually work ... erm, by limiting
variety. Whether it's the grapefruit die... soup diet, the
rice diet, or the ice cream diet, restricting ... all list of
acceptable foods helps to avoid the renewed ... es
with sensory variety. After all, there's just so muc...
even ice cream, any normal person would ever want ...

If you restrict variety, you'll eat less. But it's a short
effect. Eventually, our desire for more eating choices wins ot
sometimes in calorie-busting ways. Why? One reason is "mono...
effects." This is different from sensory-specific satiety, which is a
short-term phenomenon, often affecting just the foods at one meal.
Monotony effects refer to the boredom we experience with a food
when we eat it meal after meal or even day after day. Such monotony effects are not seen with every food—there are some foods we
eat every day with enjoyment. For example, we never seem to tire
of some staples such as bread, cereals, potatoes, and dairy products,
as well as tea and coffee. Other highly palatable foods, like potato
chips or chocolate, are subject to sensory-specific satiety, but not
monotony: If you like potato chips, you may tire of them after a
while at one meal, but the next day, they're just as attractive.

The foods we do tire of when we eat them repeatedly are those
that make up the main component of a meal, such as meat, or foods
with a high-fat content. So, for example, if you had lasagna yester-
day you may not want it today or even for several weeks, but
shrimp that you last tried at a wedding a month ago will be very
appealing.

So restricting variety may work for a brief period of time, but eventually, over weeks, you'll just want the foods you're not allowing yourself even more. What to do? The latest research [...] more attention to just what kinds of foods we're making [...] It goes back to the core concept of this book: If [...] more calories than you need, you'll want to cha[nge the ener]gy density of your overall eating naturally, to feel full witho[ut ...]at. But what does this have to do with sensory-s[...] Quite a bit, as it turns out.

When [...] satiety for a specific food, it's not the calori[...] the portion size. As long as you eat a nor[mal ...] you'll get enough sensory stimulation to trigger [...] satiety. Eat a standard portion of a food that's been calorie energy density, and sensory-specific-satiety will kick in [at a lo]wer calorie level. This is one of the ways that energy density [inf]luences satiety.

MAKE VARIETY YOUR ALLY

The latest research finds that both normal-weight and overweight people look for variety in what they eat. But the kinds of variety they seek are very different. A study at Tufts University in Boston finds that overweight people eat a wide variety of energy-dense foods. *Normal-weight people eat a variety of foods that are lower in energy density.*

"Eating a variety of foods that are high in energy density was associated with greater body fatness," says Tufts researcher Megan A. McCrory. She found that people who had the greatest variety of energy-dense sweets, snacks, condiments, carbohydrate-rich foods, and lunch and dinner entrees had the most body fat. "It's better to have only one kind of cookie rather than three different kinds in your cookie drawer," she says. "If you have only one kind of cookie, sensory-specific satiety tells us you are more likely to get tired of it than if you have several different kinds from which to choose. So much variety is available today that it's easy to go overboard."

That's how variety can trip you up: If you have lunch at a salad bar with fifteen different high-fat mixed dishes, it's easy to overeat. If, when you get home, you can choose between four different kinds of chips on your shelf, or between cheese-and-crackers, salami, pretzels, chips, peanut butter, or candy bars, then your variety instinct will lead you from one high-energy food to another. You'll simply eat more foods that provide calories quickly. In the end, you'll eat more calories each day, which will make weight control difficult.

The answer isn't to limit variety, which is healthful: Recent large-scale studies have found that people who eat the least varied diets are the most likely to suffer from heart disease and cancer. No wonder the Japanese nutritional guidelines encourage people to eat thirty different foods a day! Some scientists even believe that the greater variety in the French diet—they eat more vegetables than Americans, for example—may be part of the explanation for why the French have less heart disease despite eating as much saturated fat as Americans.

The real solution for both weight management and health is to *increase* the variety of low energy-dense foods around you. In the Tufts study, the food category most associated with lower body weight was vegetables. The greater the variety of vegetables people ate, the less they weighed. It was almost a protective effect: People who ate a wider variety of vegetables weighed less, even if they also had a wide variety of more energy-dense foods. Vegetables are just one food that's low in energy density. We already know that eating meals that are lower in energy density lead to people eating fewer calories.

So welcome variety into your life, but use it to encourage a diet with healthful foods that are lower in energy density. Think about it: What happens when you are surrounded by a wide variety of foods that are low in energy density? You'll be more likely to find a food for which you are "in the mood." After you have eaten as much as you want of that food, you'll find another low-energy-dense food that is now a little more attractive than the first one—that's the sensory-specific satiety effect. So you'll find yourself filling up on foods that provide taste and nutrition with only a modest amount of calories.

That's key. After all, it's okay if our desire for variety causes us to eat more—as long as we're eating low-energy-dense apples, strawberries, baby carrots, tomatoes, baked potato, three-bean salad, skim milk, oatmeal, tomato soup, chicken stir-fry, pasta primavera, low-fat yogurt. If you want to control your hunger without overeating, surround yourself with a wide variety of low-energy-dense foods. The more *Volumetric* foods you have around, the greater the likelihood that you'll find something you like—maybe something you haven't had for a while, something you will really enjoy for the very reason that you haven't had it recently.

SUMMARY

- As we eat a food, it becomes less pleasant until we experience satiety for it. But we'll enjoy another food with different sensory attributes. That's sensory-specific satiety.

- Taste, aroma, texture, color, and shape each affect satiety. Varying the sensory attributes of different courses can increase how much we eat by as much as 60 percent.

- To guard against overeating, chew your food fully, savoring its flavor, texture, and aroma. Look for foods that give you sensory stimulation for a long time with few calories.

- At buffets, cafeterias, and salad bars, where tremendous choice is offered, fill your plate with low-calorie salad greens and veggies with a small amount of dressing, and then take small portions of a number of other foods.

- Rather than attempting to manage the variety effect with a boring, restrictive diet—a strategy that will backfire—make variety your ally. Surround yourself with a wide selection of enjoyable foods that are low in energy density. That way, as one *Volumetric* food becomes less attractive, there will be another one that you'll want to eat.

Sizing Up Portions

"What kind of sandwich isn't fattening?"
"Half a sandwich."
—CONVERSATION BETWEEN JELLY AND ANOTHER
GANGSTER IN THE MOVIE *Analyze This*

AT THE UNIVERSITY OF GOETTINGEN in Germany in the late
1970s, obesity researchers devised a study worthy of *Candid Camera*. For 3 days, they served people soup from normal bowls, so
they could determine each person's customary intake. On the fourth
day, without telling anyone, they substituted a trick bowl that very
slowly refilled itself from a hidden reservoir under the table so that
it was never empty.

Everyone ate at least a third more soup.

Some people ate two-thirds more.

You don't have to sip from a trick bowl to eat more. Portion
sizes in the United States are expanding at an astounding rate, and
large portions encourage overeating.

VOLUMETRIC PORTIONS

What does this have to do with energy density?

Everything.

If your diet consists of lots of high-fat and energy-dense foods,
you'll have to eat smaller portions to cut calories, and that's very
hard to do. The amount of food you can eat to lose weight or even
to avoid gaining weight will be too small to satisfy your hunger. It's
only by lowering the energy density of your overall dietary pattern
that you can maintain satisfying portions. For foods of very low
energy density, such as most fruits and vegetables, you may need to
eat portions that are *bigger* than what's usual for you. For these
foods, portion size is much less important.

But you will still need to watch portion sizes carefully for those energy-dense foods you want to include in your life. If you eat nuts or cheese or chips until you are full, you'll take in too many calories. To satisfy hunger, you'll want to fill up on *Volumetric* foods of lower energy density first. Then, when you eat high-calorie foods, you can enjoy small portions.

RISING PORTIONS

The United States Department of Agriculture defines the "serving size" of the basic foods in the Food Guide Pyramid (see p. 111). These are smaller than the portions that most people eat. When New York University's Lisa Young asked nutrition students to bring in a "medium" bagel, baked potato, muffin, or cookie, for example, the amounts they brought were more than double USDA serving sizes. The average muffin was 5.2 ounces—more than 3 muffin servings. "People think that what they eat is a serving no matter how big it is," says Young. The caloric effects can be huge. A plain 2-ounce bagel has 150 calories, but that means if yours is 6 ounces, it's 450 calories, and that's before you put anything on it!

Portions are growing, too. Restaurant pasta bowls hold more than 2 pounds. A plate of steak or fish that weighs more than a pound is no longer unusual restaurant fare. In a movie house, a "medium" popcorn holds 16 cups (with up to 1,000 calories). A serving size of ice cream is ½ cup, but in restaurants, a "scoop" is 1½ to 2 cups. "Since the early 1980s, there has been a trend toward bigger portions—and bigger people," says Young. Says New York University's Marion Nestle, "Big portions sell foods, but it means that people are confronted by more food than they need."

BIG PACKAGES ENCOURAGE MORE EATING

Economy packages may save you money but they cost you calories. So finds Brian Wansink, of the University of Illinois at Champaign-Urbana:

- **Spaghetti.** When Wansink gave women a 2-pound box of spaghetti and asked them to take out enough to make a dinner for two, they pulled an average of 302 strands. But when he gave them a 1-pound box, they removed only 234 strands.

- **Cooking oil.** When asked to fry a chicken dinner for two, women poured 4.3 ounces from a 32-ounce bottle, but only 3.5 ounces from a 16-ounce bottle.

- **Candy.** When Wansink asked people to show him how many M&M's they would eat while watching a movie by themselves, participants poured 63 from a small package that contained 114 candies, 103 from a package double in size, and 122 from a package triple in size. That is, they selected about twice as much from a jumbo bag, a difference of about 250 calories.

- **Movie popcorn.** In a Chicago movie theater, Wansink gave consumers either small (about 4 ounces) or large (8 ounces) buckets of popcorn. When they got the large buckets, they ate 46 percent more. That was true for men who saw the movie with men, and women who saw the movie with women. But there was one exception: women on dates. They were not influenced by package size.

"Bigger packages are more convenient and offer tremendous cost savings," says Wansink, "but you may end up eating 40 percent to 50 percent more."

IF YOU SERVE IT, THEY WILL EAT

Sitting down to large portions on your plate also encourages overeating. There is a strong tendency for people to try to finish all the food on their plates. Many adults were taught by their parents to do this at an early age. Obese individuals are particularly prone to clean the plate, research shows.

We've found that even lean young men, who in general regulate their food intake well, ate more when they were given bigger portions. We offered them a macaroni and cheese lunch on three separate occasions. When we gave them 16 ounces, they ate 10 ounces. When we gave them 22 ounces, they ate 13 ounces. When we gave them a "jumbo" plate of 25 ounces, they ate 15 ounces, that is, 50 percent more than when they were given the 16-ounce portion.

Because big portion sizes encourage overeating, the decisions of food servers can have a big impact on your food intake. So you had better not rely on someone else to serve you an appropriate amount of food. Many chefs rely on experience and tradition, rather than calorie or nutrient content, when deciding portion size.

HELP YOURSELF

Here are some ways to prevent supersize portions from stimulating overeating:

- **Shopping.** If you purchase energy-dense snack foods such as chips or cookies, buy the smallest package. You might even look for individually wrapped portions. Or buy large packages for economy, and then transfer the contents into smaller sealable plastic bags or storage containers. For staple foods, such as oil, you can also buy big cheaper packages, but when you get home, transfer the contents to smaller bottles.

- **Cooking.** When making large batches of foods that can be frozen, portion them out into single-serving freezer/microwave containers, so you can make a quick portion-controlled meal in minutes.

- **Eating at home.** When people serve themselves, they tend to eat about the same weight of food, so it is important that you reduce the energy density of frequently eaten foods. If someone else serves the food, make sure that the portions are appropriate for your calorie level. You may also want to try smaller plates, so portions look more substantial.

- **Eating out.** In a sit-down restaurant, check the menu or ask the waiter if small or half-size portions are available. If you find you are served a big portion, remember it is okay to leave food on your plate. If you can't stand waste, ask to have leftovers wrapped to take home. Alternately, you might order just an appetizer and a salad, or share an entree with your dining partner. In a fast-food restaurant, choose small portions, including beverages.

SUMMARY

- Energy density and portion sizes are intimately linked. If you lower the energy density of frequently eaten foods, you can eat larger portions without increasing calories.

- For foods of low energy density, portion size is relatively unimportant. To enjoy energy-dense foods such as sweets, snacks, cheeses, nuts, and certain meats without overeating, however, you'll need to monitor portions carefully.

- Large packages purchased in supermarkets, and large portions served in restaurants, encourage overeating.

- Learn appropriate serving sizes, and practice portion-size self-defense: When shopping, purchase small packages or repack foods in small containers at home.

- At home, store foods in individual portions. When eating out, order less, and if you get too much, decide on an appropriate portion, and leave the rest or take it home.

Meal Timing Myths: Questions and Answers

All happiness depends upon a leisurely breakfast.
—JOHN GUNTHER, *Newsweek*, 1970

PEOPLE WHO ARE TRYING TO LOSE WEIGHT are often advised to change not only what they eat, but *how* they eat. These are satiety strategies. But many common ones haven't been shown to be effective. It's hard enough to make changes in what you eat without making changes in how you eat that don't work!

Should I eat more slowly?

It's not necessary. The idea is that pausing between bites, chewing slowly, and taking smaller bites will help you control your eating and allow time for satiety mechanisms to be activated. But it hasn't been shown to work; in one study, people who paused between bites actually wound up eating more! Even in weight loss programs where it seemed to help initially, the effect didn't last after several months.

Our advice: Eat at a pace that maximizes your enjoyment. If slowing down and savoring the flavors and textures of foods leaves you feeling more satisfied, go for it. It's true that satiety signals take time to be experienced, so after you've eaten an amount of food that should be satisfying, you may want to wait 15 or 20 minutes before deciding whether you are still hungry. But don't put a lot of effort into techniques like putting down your fork every time you take a bite.

Is skipping meals okay?

It's not wise to skip meals. When you skip meals, you are likely to overcompensate by eating more at the next meal. You'll consume more total calories.

Should I eat breakfast?

Yes. Breakfast skippers are especially prone to weight gain (see "Breakfast Benefits," p. 67).

Will frequent small meals help me control hunger?

Only if you make the right food choices. Theoretically, eating several small meals a day rather than one or two big ones helps stabilize the way the body burns fuel, avoiding the big calorie boosts that are easy for the body to turn into body fat. But this way of eating hasn't been shown to help people burn calories better, or to help with weight loss. What's more, for many people, eating more frequently means eating more snacks, which are commonly high in energy density.

Watch what you eat, not how often. If you find that eating more frequently helps control hunger, that's great. Most people eat around five times a day with two additional beverage breaks. If your current pattern works for you, there's no need to change it for weight management.

Should I snack?

Snacking per se is not linked with obesity, but your choice of snack matters. A pattern of eating high-fat, high-energy-dense foods for snacks has been shown to bump up the proportion of fat in your diet, which can lead to weight gain. Soft drinks between meals also add extra calories to your daily total. Most kids snack frequently because they need the extra calories, but if you keep the habit as an adult, you need to choose snacks of lower energy density. If you mindlessly munch on high-calorie foods as you drive to work or back home, if you keep high-fat, energy-dense snacks for impulsive munching at your desk, or if you nibble to alleviate stress, you'll undermine your weight management goals. (For smart snack choices, see 100-Calorie Snacks, p. 298.)

Should I avoid eating after 8 p.m.?

This is another myth. In a large survey of 1,800 Americans, there was no association between the extent of evening eating and weight change over a 10-year period. When the USDA's Nancy Keim gave overweight women 70 percent of their calories either before noon or after 4:30 in the afternoon for 12 weeks, it made no difference in the amount of body fat. "We didn't study whether people eat more high-fat foods like pizza and buttered popcorn later in the evening," admits Keim. But that only reinforces the point: Focus on food choices, not timing. "So many diet strategies in the popular press say don't eat after 6 p.m. or 8 p.m., but our culture may not lend itself to that—many people may not have time to eat before then, says Keim. I don't want anyone to say, 'Oh, my time has elapsed, I can't eat.' When you eat is not as critical as the quality of the foods you are selecting."

100-Calorie Snacks

For weight management, it doesn't matter whether you snack, but it *does* matter what you snack on. If you choose wisely, you can fill up on a snack of only 100 calories:

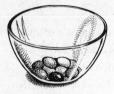 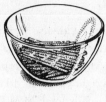 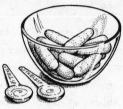

Jelly beans.
E.D.: 3.7.
Serving size: 1 ounce
(10 large beans).

Fat-free pretzel twists.
E.D.: 3.6.
Serving size: 1 ounce
(18 tiny pretzels).

Baby carrots with
fat-free dressing.
E.D.: 0.6. Serving size:
12 carrots and 2 table-
spoons dressing.

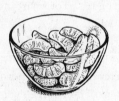 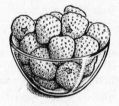

Orange sections.
E.D.: 0.5.
Serving size: 1 ¼ cups.

Strawberries.
E.D.: 0.2. Serving size:
2 ¾ cups.

Resources and
References

Resources

THE FOLLOWING RESOURCES PROVIDE sound information on nutrition, weight loss, and physical activity.

GENERAL NUTRITION INFORMATION

American Dietetic Association

The largest association for nutrition professionals in the United States. Provides responsible nutrition information. Can help you find a Registered Dietitian (R.D.) in your area. (800) 366–1655. (9 A.M.–4 P.M. Central Standard Time) for its Consumer Nutrition Hot Line. Web site: www.eatright.org

AMA Health Insight

A broad health site with usable nutrition information. The "Personal Nutritionist" will assess your diet and give you tips for improvement. You can also calculate your BMI easily and will be given tips on increasing your activity level. There are even recipes.
Web site: www.ama-assn.org/consumer.htm

Center for Science in the Public Interest

A nonprofit consumer advocacy group with a strong focus on nutrition; publishes the newsletter *Nutrition Action*. (202) 332-6718. Web site: www.cspinet.org

Consumer Information Center

Pueblo, CO 81009
Provides information on the many free (or inexpensive) government-prepared brochures on health, diet, and nutrition. You can view the text on the Web. Order on-line or at the address above.
Web site: www.pueblo.gsa.gov

Healthfinder

This site is sponsored by the Department of Health and Human Services. It organizes and links to health and nutrition information from a vast array of agencies and Web sites. Web site: www.healthfinder.gov

IFIC (International Food and Information Council)

This food industry–sponsored site provides scientific information on controversial topics in nutrition and food safety. Web site: www.ificinfo.health.org

Mayo Clinic Health Oasis

Provides a wide range of health information. Click on "Nutrition" and you can get advice on weight loss and healthy recipes. Shows you how to make your recipes healthy, will quiz you on your nutrition knowledge, and has a library of diet and nutrition information. Web site: www.mayohealth.org

PubMed

This is the site where both scientists and journalists keep track of the scientific literature. Anyone can use this site to tap into MEDLINE, which provides abstracts of original research articles. If you want to check out what research has been done on a particular topic or what an individual scientist has published, this site will provide that. Web site: www.ncbi.nlm.nih.gov/PubMed

Tufts University Nutrition Navigator

This is one place to start a Web search. This site rates the quality and ease of use of hundreds of nutrition-related Web sites. Web site: www.navigator.tufts.edu

USDA Food and Nutrition Information Center

This will connect you to the resources of the National Agricultural Library. It gives you information on food composition, the dietary guidelines, and the Food Guide Pyramid. It links you to other nutrition and weight control Web sites. Web site: www.nal.usda.gov/fnic

American Obesity Association (AOA)

1250 24th Street, N.W., Suite 300
Washington, DC 20037
(800) 986–2373
An advocacy group aimed at educating the public about obesity, protecting
the rights of the obese, and promoting research related to preventing or
curing obesity. You can show your support by joining this organization.
Web site: www.obesity.org

The LEARN Education Center

P.O. Box 610430, Department 70
Dallas, TX 75261–0430
(800) 736–7323
LEARN is a sound weight management program that combines diet, exer-
cise, and behavior modification. The site provides useful weight loss tips.
Web site: www.learneducation.com

National Heart, Lung and Blood Institute

This site contains general information related to cardiovascular disease.
If you want more information on the new government guidelines on overweight and obesity, you can obtain that here. Web site: www.nhlbi.nih.gov/

Weight-control Information Network (WIN)
(Part of the National Institutes of Health)

1 WIN Way
Bethesda, MD 20892–3665
(301) 984–7378 or (800) WIN–8098
Fax: (301) 984–7196
Provides science-based information on obesity. You can obtain free fact
sheets and brochures and a list of university-based weight control programs. Web site: www.niddk.nih.gov/health/nutrit/win.htm

RECIPES AND MENUS

CyberDiet's Home Page

This award-winning site has a huge amount of diet and nutrition information. You can calculate your BMI, work out a personal menu plan, and figure out how many calories your activities are burning. The menu plan comes with recipes and a shopping list and can be designed around the number of calories you want to eat.
Web site: www.cyberdiet.com

Meals for You

This site has thousands of recipes, and you can access them according to how you want to eat: for weight loss, vegetarian, low-fat, gourmet, and so on. It gives you nutritional breakdowns and preparation times. Recipes automatically adjust for number of servings and give you a shopping list.
Web site: www.MealsForYou.com

FITNESS AND PHYSICAL ACTIVITY

Shape Up America

Former Surgeon General C. Everett Koop started this campaign to reduce obesity and increase fitness. The site has up-to-date information on weight management, healthy eating, and physical fitness. It helps you to develop a fun and effective activity program. Web site: www.shapeup.org

References

PART 1: WHAT IS *VOLUMETRICS*?

The Energy Density Breakthrough

Bell, E. A., Castellanos, V. H., Pelkman, C. L., Thorwart, M. L., and Rolls, B. J. 1998. Energy density of foods affected energy intake in normal-weight women. *American Journal of Clinical Nutrition*, 67, 412–420.

Bell, E. A., Denlinger, B. A., Thorwart, M. L. and Rolls, B. J. 1999. Increasing volume of food with air affects satiety. *Obesity Research*, 7, 44S.

Duncan, K. H., Bacon, J. A., and Weinsier, R. L. 1983. The effects of high and low energy density diets on satiety, energy intake, and eating time of obese and nonobese subjects. *American Journal of Clinical Nutrition*, 37, 763–767.

Fitzwater, S. L., Weinsier, R. L., Wooldridge, N. H., Birch, R., Liu, C., and Bartolucci, A. A. 1991. Evaluation of long-term weight changes after a multidisciplinary weight control program. *Journal of the American Dietetic Association*, 91, 421–426, 429.

Poppitt, S. D. 1995. Energy density of diets and obesity. *International Journal of Obesity*, 19, S20-S26.

Prentice, A. M. 1998. Manipulation of dietary fat and energy density and subsequent effects on substrate flux and food intake. *American Journal of Clinical Nutrition*, 67, 535S–541S.

Rolls, B. J., and Bell, E. A. 1999. Intake of fat and carbohydrate: Role of energy density. *European Journal of Clinical Nutrition*, 52, 1–8.

Rolls, B. J., Bell, E. A., Castellanos, V. H., Chow, M., Pelkman, C. L., and Thorwart, M. L. 1999. Energy density but not fat content of foods affected energy intake in lean and obese women. *American Journal of Clinical Nutrition*, 69, 863–871.

Saltzman, E., Dallal, G. E., and Roberts, S. B. 1997. Effect of high-fat and low-fat diets on voluntary energy intake and substrate oxidation: Studies in identical twins consuming diets matched for energy density, fiber and palatability. *American Journal of Clinical Nutrition*, 66, 1332–1339.

Strain, G. W., Hershcopf, R. J., and Zumoff, B. 1992. Food intake of very obese persons: Quantitative and qualitative aspects. *Journal of the American Dietetic Association*, 92, 199–203.

Stubbs, R. J., Johnstone, A. M., O'Reilly, L. M., Barton, K., and Reid, C. 1998. The effect of covertly manipulating the energy density of mixed diets on ad libitum food intake in "pseudo free-living" humans. *International Journal of Obesity*, 22, 980–987.

Stubbs, R. J., Ritz, P., Coward, W. A., and Prentice, A. M. 1995. Covert manipulation of the ratio of dietary fat to carbohydrate and energy density: Effect on food intake and energy balance in free-living men eating ad libitum. *American Journal of Clinical Nutrition*, 62, 330–337.

van Stratum, P., Lussenburg, R. N., van Wezel, L. A., Vergroesen, A. J., and Cremer, H. D. 1978. The effect of dietary carbohydrate: Fat ratio on energy intake by adult women. *American Journal of Clinical Nutrition*, 31, 206–212.

PART 2: HOW TO LOSE WEIGHT AND KEEP IT OFF

Creating Your Own Weight Management Program

Foreyt, J. P., and Poston, W. S. C. II. 1998. The role of the behavioral counselor in obesity treatment. *Journal of the American Dietetic Association*, 98, S27-S30.

Foster, G. D., Wadden, T. A., Vogt, R. A., and Brewer, G. 1997. What is a reasonable weight loss? Patients' expectations and evaluations of obesity treatment outcomes. *Journal of Consulting and Clinical Psychology*, 65, 79–85.

National Institutes of Health. National Heart, Lung, and Blood Institute. *Clinical Guidelines on the Identification, Evaluation, and Treatment of Overweight and Obesity in Adults*. U.S. Department of Health and Human Services, 1998.

Shick, S. M., Wing, R. R., Klem, M. L., McGuire, M. T., Hill, J. O., and Seagle, H. 1998. Persons successful at long-term weight loss and maintenance continue to consume a low-energy, low-fat diet. *Journal of the American Dietetic Association*, 98, 408–413.

Fat

American Dietetic Association. 1998. Position of the American Dietetic Association: Fat replacers. *Journal of the American Dietetic Association*, 98, 463–468.

Castellanos, V. H., and Rolls, B. J. Diet composition and the regulation of food intake and body weight. In *Overweight and Weight Management*, ed. S. Dalton. Aspen, 1997: 254–83.

Cheskin, L. J., Miday, R., Zorich, N., and Filloon, T. 1998. Gastrointestinal symptoms following consumption of olestra or regular triglyceride potato chips: A controlled comparison. *Journal of the American Medical Association*, 279 (2), 150–152.

Drewnowski, A. 1997. Why do we like fat? *Journal of the American Dietetic Association*, 97 (7 Suppl.), S58-S62.

Hill, J. O., Drougas, H., and Peters, J. C. 1993. Obesity treatment: Can diet composition play a role? *Annals of Internal Medicine*, 119, 694–697.

Kristal, A. R., White, E., Shattuck, A. L., Curry, S., Anderson, G. L., Fowler, A., and Urban, N. 1992. Long-term maintenance of a low-fat diet: Durability of fat-related dietary habits in the Women's Health Trial. *Journal of the American Dietetic Association*, 92, 553–559.

Lissner, L., Heitmann, B. L., and Bengtsson, C. 1997. Low-fat diets may prevent weight gain in sedentary women: Prospective observations from the population study of women in Gothenburg, Sweden. *Obesity Research*, 5, 43–48.

Peterson, S., Sigman-Grant, M., Eissenstat, B., and Kris-Etherton, P. 1999. Impact of adopting lower-fat food choices on energy and nutrient intakes of American adults. *Journal of the American Dietetic Association*, 99, 177–183.

Rolls, B. J. 1997. Fat and sugar substitutes and the control of food intake. *Annals of the New York Academy of Sciences*, 819, 180–193.

Rolls, B. J., and Hammer, V. A. 1995. Fat, carbohydrate and the regulation of energy intake. *American Journal of Clinical Nutrition*, 62, 1086S–1095S.

Carbohydrates

American Dietetic Association. 1998. Position of the American Dietetic Association: Use of nutritive and nonnutritive sweeteners. *Journal of the American Dietetic Association*, 98, 580–587.

Astrup, A., and Raben, A. 1995. Carbohydrate and obesity. *International Journal of Obesity*, 19, S27-S37.

Blackburn, G. L., Kanders, B. S., Lavin, P. T., Keller, S. D., and Whatley, J. 1997. The effect of aspartame as part of a multidisciplinary weight-control program on short- and long-term control of body weight. *American Journal of Clinical Nutrition*, 65, 409–418.

Golay, A., Allaz, Anne-F., Morel, Y., de Tonnac, N., Tankova, S., and Reaven, G. 1996. Similar weight loss with low- or high-carbohydrate diets. *American Journal of Clinical Nutrition*, 63, 174–178.

Hill, J. O., and Prentice, A. M. 1995. Sugar and body weight regulation. *American Journal of Clinical Nutrition*, 62, 264S–274S.

Levine, A. S., and Billington, C. J. Dietary fiber: Does it affect food intake and body weight? In *Appetite and Body Weight Regulation: Sugar, Fat, and Macronutrient Substitutes*, eds. J. D. Fernstrom and G. D. Miller, CRC Press, Inc., 1994: 191–200.

Pasman, W. J., Westerterp-Plantenga, M. S., Muls, E., Vansant, G., van Ree, J., and Saris, W. H. M. 1997. The effectiveness of long-term fibre supplementation on weight maintenance in weight-reduced women. *International Journal of Obesity*, 21, 548–555.

Raben, A., Macdonald, I., and Astrup, A. 1997. Replacement of dietary fat by sucrose or starch: Effects on 14d ad libitum energy intake, energy expenditure and body weight in formerly obese and never-obese subjects. *International Journal of Obesity*, 21, 846–859.

Rolls, B. J. 1991. Effects of intense sweeteners on hunger, food intake and body weight: A review. *American Journal of Clinical Nutrition*, 53, 872–878.

Rolls, B. J., and Hill, J. O. 1998. *Carbohydrates and Weight Management*. ILSI Press.

Schlundt, D. G., Hill, J. O., Sbrocco, T., Pope-Cordle, J., and Sharp, T. 1992. The role of breakfast in the treatment of obesity: A randomized clinical trial. *American Journal of Clinical Nutrition*, 55(3), 645–651.

Surwit, R. S., Feinglos, M. N., McCaskill, C. C., Clay, S. L., Babyak, M. A., Brownlow, B. S., Plaisted, C. S., and Lin, Pao-H. 1997. Metabolic and behavioral effects of a high-sucrose diet during weight loss. *American Journal of Clinical Nutrition*, 65, 908–915.

Protein

Barkeling, B., Rossner, S., and Bjorvell, H. 1990. Effects of a high-protein meal (meat) and a high-carbohydrate meal (vegetarian) on satiety measured by automated computerized monitoring of subsequent food intake, motivation to eat and food preferences. *International Journal of Obesity*, 14, 743–751.

Doucet, E., and Tremblay, A. 1997. Food intake, energy balance and body weight control. *European Journal of Clinical Nutrition*, 51, 846–855.

Nelson, L. H., and Tucker, L. A. 1996. Diet composition related to body fat in a multivariate study of 203 men. *Journal of the American Dietetic Association*, 96, 771–777.

Poppitt, S. D., McCormack, D., and Buffenstein, R. 1998. Short-term effects of macronutrient preloads on appetite and energy intake in lean women. *Physiology and Behavior*, 64, 279–285.

Rolls, B. J., Hetherington, M., and Burley, V. J. 1988. The specificity of satiety: The influence of foods of different macronutrient content on the development of satiety. *Physiology and Behavior*, 43, 145–153.

Stubbs, R. J., van Wyk, M. C. W., Johnstone, A. M., and Harbron, C. G. 1996. Breakfasts high in protein, fat or carbohydrate: Effect on within-day appetite and energy balance. *European Journal of Clinical Nutrition*, 50, 409–417.

Uhe, A. M., Collier, G. R., and O'Dea, K. 1992. A comparison of the effects of beef, chicken and fish protein on satiety and amino acid profiles in lean male subjects. *Journal of Nutrition*, 122, 467–472.

Alcohol

de Castro, J. M., and Orozco, S. 1990. Moderate alcohol intake and spontaneous eating patterns of humans: Evidence of unregulated supplementation. *American Journal of Clinical Nutrition*, 52, 246–253.

Foltin, R. W., Kelly, T. H., and Fischman, M. W. 1993. Ethanol as an energy source in humans: Comparison with dextrose-containing beverages. *Appetite*, 20, 95–110.

Murgatroyd, P. R., Van De Ven, M. L. H. M., Goldberg, G. R., and Prentice, A. M. 1996. Alcohol and the regulation of energy balance: Overnight effects on diet-induced thermogenesis and fuel storage. *British Journal of Nutrition*, 75, 33–45.

Poppitt, S. D., Eckhardt, J. W., McGonagle, J., Murgatroyd, P. R., and Prentice, A. M. 1996. Short-term effects of alcohol consumption on appetite and energy intake. *Physiology and Behavior*, 60, 1063–1070.

Prentice, A. M. 1995. Alcohol and obesity. *International Journal of Obesity*, 19, (Supplement 5) S44-S50.

Tremblay, A., Wouters, E., Wenker, M., St-Pierre, S., Bouchard, C., and Despres, Jean-P. 1995. Alcohol and a high-fat diet: A combination favoring overfeeding. *American Journal of Clinical Nutrition*, 62, 639–644.

Westerterp-Plantenga, M. S., and Verwegen, C. R. T. 1999. The appetizing effect of an aperitif in overweight and normal-weight humans. *American Journal of Clinical Nutrition*, 69, 205–212.

Water and Other Beverages

Bolton, R. P., Heaton, K. W., and Burroughs, L. F. 1981. The role of dietary fiber in satiety, glucose, and insulin: Studies with fruit and fruit juice. *American Journal of Clinical Nutrition*, 34, 211–217.

de Castro, J. M. 1993. The effects of the spontaneous ingestion of particular foods or beverages on the meal pattern and overall nutrient intake of humans. *Physiology and Behavior*, 53, 1133–1144.

Kleiner, S. M. 1999. Water: An essential but overlooked nutrient. *Journal of the American Dietetic Association*, 99, 200–206.

Jacobson, Michael F. *Liquid Candy: How Soft Drinks Are Harming Americans' Health*. Center for Science in the Public Interest, 1998.

Rolls, B. J., Castellanos, V. H., Halford, J. C., Kilara, A., Panyam, D., Pelkman, C. L., Smith, G. P., and Thorwart, M. L. 1998. Volume of Food consumed affects satiety in men. *American Journal of Clinical Nutrition*, 67, 1170–1177.

Rolls, B. J., Fedoroff, I. C., Guthrie, J. F., and Laster, L. J. 1990. Effects of temperature and mode of presentation of juice on hunger, thirst and food intake in humans. *Appetite*, 15, 199–208.

Rolls, B. J., Kim, S., and Fedoroff, I. C. 1990. Effects of drinks sweetened with sucrose or aspartame on hunger, thirst and food intake in men. *Physiology and Behavior*, 48, 19–26.

Tordoff, M. G., and Alleva, A. M. 1990. Effect of drinking soda sweetened with aspartame or high-fructose corn syrup on food intake and body weight. *American Journal of Clinical Nutrition*, 51, 963–969.

Soup

Foreyt, J. P., Reeves, R. S., Darnell, L. S., Wohlleb, J. C., and Gotto, A. M. 1986. Soup consumption as a behavioral weight loss strategy. *Journal of the American Dietetic Association*, 86, 524–526.

Himaya, A., and Louis-Sylestre, J. 1998. The effect of soup on satiation. *Appetite*, 30, 199–210.

Jordan, H. A., Levitz, L. S., Utgoff, K. L., and Lee, H. L. 1981. Role of food characteristics in behavioral change and weight loss. *Journal of the American Dietetic Association*, 79, 24–29.

Rolls, B. J., Bell, E. A., and Thorwart, M. L. 1999. Water incorporated into a food but not served with a food decreases energy intake in lean women. *American Journal of Clinical Nutrition*, 70, 448–455.

Rolls, B. J., Fedoroff, I. C., Guthrie, J. F., and Laster, L. J. 1990. Foods with different satiating effects in humans. *Appetite*, 15, 115–126.

PART 4: THE FOOD GUIDE

U. S. Department of Agriculture Human Nutrition Information Service, The Food Guide Pyramid, 1992, *Home & Garden Bulletin* #252.

First Data Bank Inc., Nutritionist Five [computer software]. San Bruno, Calif, 1998.

PART 6: AN ACTIVE LIFE

The Exercise Prescription

Andersen, R. E., Wadden, T. A., Bartlett, S. J., Zemel, B., Verde, T. J., and Franckowiak, S. C. 1999. Effects of lifestyle activity vs. structured aerobic exercise in obese women. *Journal of the American Medical Association*, 281, 335–340.

Doucet, E., and Tremblay, A. 1998. Body weight loss and maintenance with physical activity and diet. *Coronary Artery Disease*, 9, 495–501.

Hills, A. P., and Byrne, N. M. 1998. Exercise prescription for weight management. *Proceedings of the Nutrition Society*, 57, 93–103.

Horton, T. J., and Hill, J. O. 1998. Exercise and obesity. *Proceedings of the Nutrition Society*, 57, 85–91.

King, N. A. 1998. The relationship between physical activity and food intake. *Proceedings of the Nutrition Society*, 57, 77–84.

Salzman, E., and Roberts, S. B. 1995. The role of energy expenditure in energy regulation: Findings from a decade of research. *Nutrition Reviews*, 95, 209–220.

Tremblay, A., Doucet, E., and Imbeault, P. 1999. Physical activity and weight maintenance. *International Journal of Obesity*, 23, S50–54.

PART 7: THE SATIETY LIFESTYLE

Are You Hungry?

Abramson, E. *Emotional Eating: What You Need to Know Before Starting Another Diet*. Jossey-Bass Publishers, 1998.

Fletcher, A. M. *Thin for Life: 10 Keys to Success from People Who Have Lost Weight and Kept It Off*. Chapters Publishers Ltd., 1994.

Foreyt, J. P., and Goodrick, G. K. *Living Without Dieting: A Revolutionary Guide for Everyone Who Wants to Lose Weight*. Warner Books, 1994.

Friedman, M. I., Ulrich, P., and Mattes, R. D. 1999. A figurative measure of subjective hunger sensations. *Appetite*, 32, 395–404.

Gibson, E. L., and Desmond, E. 1999. Chocolate craving and hunger state: Implications for the acquisition and expression of appetite and food choice. *Appetite*, 32, 219–240.

Koch, K. L. Stomach. In *Atlas of Gastrointestinal Motility in Health and Disease*. ed. M. M. Schuster, Williams & Wilkins, 1993: 158–76.

Michener, W., and Rozin, P. 1994. Pharmacological versus sensory factors in the satiation of chocolate craving. *Physiology and Behavior*, 56, 419–422.

Polivy, J. 1996. Psychological consequences of food restriction. *Journal of the American Dietetic Association*, 96, 589–592.

Rolls, B. J., Fedoroff, I. C., and Guthrie, J. F. 1991. Gender differences in eating behavior and body weight regulation. *Health Psychology*, 10, 133–142.

Rolls, B. J., and Miller, D. L. 1997. Is the low-fat message giving people a license to eat more? *Journal of the American College of Nutrition*, 16, 535–543.

Rozin, P., Dow, S., Moscovitch, M., and Rajaram, S. 1998. What causes humans to begin and end a meal? A role for memory for what has been eaten, as evidenced by a study of multiple meal eating in amnesic patients. *American Psychological Society*, 9, 392–396.

Tribole, E., and Resch, E. 1996. *Intuitive Eating: A Recovery Book for the Chronic Dieter: Rediscover the Pleasures of Eating and Rebuild Your Body Image*. St. Martin's Mass Market Paper.

Tuomisto, T., Tuomisto, M. T., Hetherington, M., and Lappalainen, R. 1998. Reasons for initiation and cessation of eating in obese men and women and the affective consequences of eating in everyday situations. *Appetite*, 30, 211–222.

Variety

Bell, E. A., Thorwart, M. L., and Rolls, B. J. 1998. Effects of energy content and volume on sensory-specific satiety. *FASEB Journal*, 12, A347.

Davis, C. M. 1928. Self selection of diet by newly weaned infants. *American Journal of Diseases in Childhood*, 36, 651–679.

Drewnowski, A., Henderson, S. A., Shore, A. B., Fischler, C., Preziosi, P., and Hercberg, S. 1996. Diet quality and dietary diversity in France: Implications for the French paradox. *Journal of the American Dietetic Association*, 96, 663–669.

McCrory, M. A., Fuss, P. J., McCallum, J. E., Yao, M., Vinken, A. G., Hays, N. P., and Roberts, S. B. 1999. Dietary variety within food groups: Association with energy intake and body fatness in men and woman. *American Journal of Clinical Nutrition*, 69, 440–447.

Rolls, B. J. 1985. Experimental analyses of the effects of variety in a meal on human feeding. *American Journal of Clinical Nutrition*, 42, 932–939.

Rolls, B. J. 1986. Sensory-specific satiety. *Nutrition Reviews*, 44, 93–101.

Rolls, E. T., and Rolls, J. H. 1997. Olfactory sensory-specific satiety in humans. *Physiology and Behavior*, 61, 461–473.

Sizing Up Portions

Rolls, B. J., Engell, D., and Birch, L. L. 2000. Serving portion size influences 5-year-old but not 3-year-old children's food intakes. *Journal of the American Dietetic Association*, 100, 232–234.

Wansink, B. 1996. Can package size accelerate usage volume? *Journal of Marketing*, 60, 1–14.

Young, L. R., and Nestle, M. 1995. Portion sizes in dietary assessment: Issues and policy implications. *Nutrition Reviews*, 53, 149–158.

Young, L. R., and Nestle, M. 1998. Variation in perceptions of a "medium" food portion: Implications for dietary guidance. *Journal of the American Dietetic Association*, 98, 458–459.

Meal Timing Myths: Questions and Answers

Bellisle, F., McDevitt, R., and Prentice, A. M. 1997. Meal frequency and energy balance. *British Journal of Nutrition*, 77, S57-S70.

Drummond, S., Crombie, N., and Kirk, T. 1996. A critique of the effects of snacking on body weight status. *European Journal of Clinical Nutrition*, 50, 779–783.

Gatenby, S. J. 1997. Eating frequency: Methodological and dietary aspects. *British Journal of Nutrition*, 77, S7-S20.

Kant, A. K., Schatzkin, A., and Ballard-Barbash, R. 1997. Evening eating and subsequent long-term weight change in a national cohort. *International Journal of Obesity*, 21, 407–412.

Keim, N. L., Van Loan, M. D., Horn, W. F., Barbieri, T. F., and Mayclin, P. L. 1997. Weight loss is greater with consumption of large morning meals and fat-free mass is preserved with large evening meals in women on a controlled weight reduction regimen. *Journal of Nutrition*, 127, 75–82.

Spiegel, T. A., Wadden, T. A., and Foster, G. D. 1991. Objective measurement of eating rate during behavioral treatment of obesity. *Behavior Therapy*, 22, 61–67.

Yeomans, M. R., Gray, R. W., Mitchell, C. J., and True, S. 1997. Independent effects of palatability and within-meal pauses on intake and appetite ratings in human volunteers. *Appetite*, 29, 61–76.

Index

water needs during, 92
weight loss and, 35, 258
weight maintenance and, 258–59
well-being and, 37
Eyton, Audrey, 62

Fast foods, energy density chart, 139–42
Fat, body
    abdominal and health risk, 28, 29
    body mass index (BMI), 27–28, 29
    waist size and health risk, 28
Fat, dietary, 40, 41–56
    amount of fat allowed at each daily
        calorie level, 43, 43
    appeal of, 45–46
    body fat, conversion to, 46, 48
    bread with or without butter, and
        amount allowed, 43, 44
    calorie intake and lower-fat diet, 48–49
    calories per gram, 12, 12, 41
    energy density, 3, 43, 44, 45
    healthful, food sources, 42
    low- or no-fat foods, water content
        and, 2
    major food sources and tips for reducing
        fat in, 47
    milk strategy, 52
    overweight people, desire for versus
        sugar, 46
    percent of diet recommended (moder-
        ately low), 8, 40, 41–42, 48
    potato, baked, with or without butter or
        sour cream, 43, 44, 45
    preference for, and food choices, 49–50
    satiety level, 45
    saturated, 42
    six ways to eat less, 50–51
    substitutes, 52–55, 53
    synthetic (olestra), 54–55
    taste of food and, 42
    trans fats, 42
    unsaturated, 42
    weight gain and, 17–18, 41
Feta Tzatziki, 191
Fiber, 62–64
    bloating and intestinal gas, 64
    chart, grams in foods, 65–66
    grams per day recommended, 8, 75
    health benefits, 59
    intake, calculating your, 63
    insoluble, 59
    leanness and intake of, 64
    satiety and, 3, 8, 64
    soluble, 59
    water needs and, 92
Fish
    Baked Red Snapper Provencale, 227

energy density spectrum, 130–32
fried, 129
portions, restaurant, 292
protein from, 8
satiety effect, 78
serving size, 115
tips on energy density, 129
water content, 3, 97
Fisher, M. F. K., 93
Fit Again: 90 Days to Lifetime Fitness for
    the Over-35 Male (Flippin), 266
Fletcher, Anne M., 271
Foltin, Richard, 87, 90
Food guide pyramid, 110–13, 111
    serving sizes, 292
Food log or journal, 36
Foreyt, John, 29, 34, 36, 37, 101, 270, 271,
    272
F-Plan Diet, The (Eyton), 62
Fred Hutchinson Cancer Research Center,
    50
Fruit, dried
    energy density, 58, 125, 126
    fiber content, 65
    portion control and, 69
    serving size, 114
Fruit, fresh
    American consumption of, 70
    amounts allowed on weight loss diet, 69
    Basic Dinner Salad with, 205
    canned in syrup, 125
    Chicken and, Salad, 226
    easy ways to add to your diet, 70–71
    energy density ratings, 15, 57, 125–26
    fiber content, 65
    100 calories or less, 178
    Red, White, and Blue Trifle, 237
    Salad, 210
    Salad Mold, 211
    serving size, 114–15
    slushes, 100-calorie, 174
    slushes, 200-calorie, 176
    smoothies, 200-calorie, 175, 177
    Soup, 193
    tips, 125
    water content, 3, 97
    whole, versus juice, 8
    yogurt, frozen with, 200-calories, 175
    yogurt, granola, honey, and, 200-
        calories, 175–76
Fruit juice, 95–96, 125
    spritzers, 96

Gallbladder disease
    and excess weight, 27
    rapid weight loss and risk, 29
Gazpacho, 194

French fries, energy density, 58, 123
Leek Soup, 198
Mediterranean-style baked, chunks, 188
portion control and, 69
quick country mashed, 188
seasoned oven-baked fries, 188
Potato or corn chips
and bean dip, 177
energy density ratings, 15, 58, 137
fat in and fat-reducing tips, 47
water content, 3
Poultry. *See also* Chicken; Turkey
energy density spectrum, 130–32
fat in and fat-reducing tips, 47
protein from, 8
serving size, 115
tips, energy density, 129
water content, 3
Pretzels
100-calorie, *298*
energy density, 11–12, 58, 137
tomato versus fat-free, 11–12
Produce for Better Health Foundation, 70
Programs, commercial, weight loss, 22, 37
Protein, 40, 76–83
American diet and, 80–81
amino acids, 78
calories per gram, 12, *12*
calculating your need daily, 81
diet, low-carbohydrate, high protein,
56–57, 60, 76–77, 78–80
energy density, various sources, 83
energy density, six choices at 150 calories compared, *82*
food sources, 40, 81
high consumption of and health, 79
low-energy-dense choices, 8
metabolic effect, 78
overweight men and intake, 79–80
percent of diet per day, recommended, 8
portions, watching, 129
satiety level, 40, 45, 76, 77–78
Volumetric choices, 82–83
weight loss strategies with, 77, 80–81,
83
Pumpkin, Baked, Custard, 245

Raisins, energy density, 11, *11*
Ranch
Creamy Cucumber, Salad Dressing,
212–13
Salsa Dip, 192
Raspberry(ies)
Three Berry Smoothie, 176
Reaven, Gerald, 60, 61
Red, White, and Blue Trifle, 237
Recipes, modifying favorite, 253–56

Reeds, Peter, 78, 79
Respiratory problems, and excess weight, 27
Rice
Calypso Chicken Packages, 223
Chicken, and Vegetable Soup, 202
energy density chart, 118–20
fiber content, chart, 66
serving size, 114
Shrimp and Vegetable Risotto, 228–29
Stir-fry, 221–22
Ricotta cheese
Lemon Cheesecake Soufflé, 244–45
Red, White, and Blue Trifle, 237
Vegetable Frittata, 250–51
Rimm, Eric, 86
Rozin, Paul, 274

Saccharin, 74
Salad dressing/mayonnaise
Caesar, 212
Citrus Vinaigrette, 213
Creamy Cucumber Ranch, 212–13
energy density ratings, 15, 142–45
fat in and fat-reducing tips, 47
lower fat, or no-fat, 53, *53*
Tomato Herb, 214
Salads
Basic Dinner, with Fruit, 205
Basic Dinner, with Vegetables, 204
Chef's, 206
Chicken and Fruit, 226
Crunchy and Creamy Potato, 207
energy density ratings, 15
Fruit, 210
Fruit, Mold, 211
Italian pasta, 200 calories, portions, *15*,
15–16
Moroccan Garden Couscous, 208
Tuna Ranch, 229
Waldorf, 209
Salsa
Huevos Rancheros, 251
Ranch, Dip, 192
Sandwiches, modifying to reduce energy
density, 253–54, *254*
Satiety, 2, 277–78
air-added or whipped foods, 17
alcohol and, 40
beverages, 97
bloating and, 279
carbohydrates and, 8, 40, 45
energy density and amount of food
eaten, 16–18
factors in, 3
fiber and, 3, 64
fish and, 78
getting in touch with, 278–80

grilled or broiled, 186
roasted, 186
sautéed, 186
Vegetable Frittata, 250–51
Sweet potato, 188
baked mashed, 188
microwave maple-flavored, 189
Peanut Chicken Stew, 225
Pork with, and Apples, 220

Tea, iced, 96
Thin for Life (Fletcher), 271
Thoughts and feelings. *See also* Overeating
cognitive restructuring and, 36–37
portions of food and, 20
Tofu
Stir-fry, 221–22
Tomato(es)
Baked Red Snapper Provencale, 227
Chili Ranchero, 218–19
energy density, 11–12
Gazpacho, 194
Herb Vinaigrette, 214
Tremblay, Angelo, 78, 87, 90
Tribole, Evelyn, 271, 272
Tuna Ranch Salad, 229
Turkey
Great American Volumetric Burger,
217–18
Roast, Soup, 202–3
Twain, Mark, 91

University of Alabama, weight loss program,
21, 69
University of Goettingen, portion experi-
ment, 291
University of Pennsylvania, weight loss
program, 25–26
University of Pittsburgh
National Weight Control Registry, 48
School of Medicine, 26

Vanderbilt University, Nashville, 67
Variety (of foods)
amount eaten and, 284–85
energy density and, 288–90
managing, 285–88
nutritional balance and, 286–87
sameness of food and loss of appetite
(monotony effect), 281–82, 287
sensory-specific satiety, 283–84
tips to control overeating and, 290
Vegetable(s)
American consumption of, 70
amounts allowed on weight loss diet, 69
Basic Dinner Salad with, 204
burger, energy density, 138

carbohydrates and, 8
Chef's Salad, 206
Chicken, Rice, and, Soup, 202
cooked, under 100 calories, 179–80
Curry Soup, 199
easy ways to add to your diet, 70–71
energy density ratings, 15, 57, 122–24
fiber content, chart, 65–66
Four-Cheese, Lasagna, 231–32
fried, 123
Frittata, 250–51
juice, 97
Light and Fresh, Soup, 196
Moroccan Garden Couscous Salad, 208
nonstarchy, 122
Omelet, 252
Pasta Primavera, 235
Quick Minestrone, 195
raw, under 30 calories, 179
recommendations on type to eat, 70
serving size, 114
Shrimp and, Risotto, 228–29
side dishes, under 100 calories, 180–86
side dishes, under 150 calories, 186–89
spaghetti dinner, 400 calorie, *69*
starchy, 122
Steak and, Kabobs, 215
Stir-fry, 221–22
tips, 122
variety, increasing, 70
water content, 3
whole, versus juice, 8
Vegetarian Burger, 232–33
Veggie Pita, 177
Vinaigrette
Citrus, 213
Tomato Herb, 214
Volumetric Pizza, 230–31
Volumetrics. See also Menus
breakfast cereal compared, 160 calories,
68
carbohydrates and, 67, 69
dieting roller coast eliminated with,
272
food guide pyramid, 110–13, *111*
health benefits immediate, 34
how it works, 20–21
hunger, getting back in touch with, 270
portions, 291–92
principles of, 8–9, 25
programs using, 21–22
protein choices, 82–83, *82*
studies on keeping volume of food but
reducing calories, 19
success of programs using approach,
21–22
water, role in, 91, 97–99

Waldorf Salad, 209
Wansink, Brian, 274, 292–93
Water, 91–99
    as beverage choice, 96
    calories per gram, 12, *12*
    content of foods, chart, 97
    energy density and, 3, 13–14, 40
    food consumption not decreased by, 93
    health benefits, 94
    high-volume foods, 3
    low-volume foods, 3, 13
    optimal consumption of, 9, 92
    satiety and, 2, 13, 91, 93
    strategies for lowering energy density of
        foods with, 98
    thirst and, 92, 93, 95
    urine color and, 92
Weight cycling (yo-yo dieting), 30
Weight loss. *See also* Exercise; Fat, dietary
    artificial sweeteners and, 74–75
    caloric deficit, creating, 4, 31
    calorie reduction per day for, 8
    calorie requirements for, how to figure,
        32–33
    changing just ½ of daily foods and, 19
    diet sodas and, 95
    energy density and, 21–22
    exercise and, 258–59
    expectations, realistic, 26
    gradual, advantages of, 4–5
    menu plan, how to use, 153–54
    menu plan overview, 150–51
    menus, 154–73
    menus, calorie levels, 151–52
    NIH recommendation on rate of loss, 30
    NIH study of methods that work, 26
    nondieting approach, 4–5, 6
    percent of body weight lost to improve
        health, 26, 28–29
    programs and social support, 37
    rapid, and health risks, 29–30
    rapid, and muscle loss, 30
    rapid, and regaining weight (yo-yo
        dieting), 30
    rapid, and slowed metabolism, 30

    seven keys to, 35–38
    soup and, 101–3
    volume of food and, 19–21
    volumetric approach at successful
        programs, 21–22
    Volumetrics way and immediate health
        benefits, 34
    weigh-in weekly, 33
Weight maintenance (keep weight off), 6–7,
        25
    calorie requirements for, how to figure,
        32–33
    exercise and, 31, 33
    gradual gain, how to prevent, 33
    high-protein diets, weight return after, 80
    lower fat diet and, 48
    NIH study of methods that work, 26
    plateaus, 31
    resuming further loss, 31
    seven keys to, 35–38
    weigh-in daily, 33
Weight Watchers, 37
    "1, 2, 3" program, 22
Weinsier, Roland I., 21, 69
Wheat germ, fiber content, 66
Winfrey, Oprah, 80
Wodehouse, P. G., 84
Women, water consumption recommended,
        9
Women's Health Trial, 48, 49–50

Yogurt
    energy density chart, 127–28
    Feta Tzatziki, 191
    frozen with fresh fruit, 200-calories, 175
    granola, honey, fruit, 200-calories,
        175–76
    Lemon Cheesecake Soufflé, 244–45
    nonfat flavored, comparison of sugar
        or aspartame, 74
    Red, White, and Blue Trifle, 237
    serving size, 115
    smoothies, 175, 176
Young, Lisa, 292
Yo-yo dieting, 30